Suicide Information for Teens

Second Edition

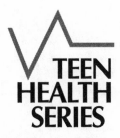

**TEEN
HEALTH
SERIES**

Second Edition

Suicide Information for Teens

Health Tips about Suicide Causes and Prevention

*Including Facts about Depression, Risk Factors,
Getting Help, Survivor Support, and More*

◆

Edited by Kim Wohlenhaus

Omnigraphics

P.O. Box 31-1640, Detroit, MI 48231

Bibliographic Note

Because this page cannot legibly accommodate all the copyright notices, the Bibliographic Note portion of the Preface constitutes an extension of the copyright notice.

Edited by Kim Wohlenhaus

Teen Health Series

Karen Bellenir, *Managing Editor*
David A. Cooke, MD, FACP, *Medical Consultant*
Elizabeth Collins, *Research and Permissions Coordinator*
Cherry Edwards, *Permissions Assistant*
EdIndex, Services for Publishers, *Indexers*

* * *

Omnigraphics, Inc.

Matthew P. Barbour, *Senior Vice President*
Kevin M. Hayes, *Operations Manager*

* * *

Peter E. Ruffner, *Publisher*
Copyright © 2010 Omnigraphics, Inc.
ISBN 978-0-7808-1088-4

Library of Congress Cataloging-in-Publication Data

Suicide information for teens : health tips about suicide causes and prevention : including facts about depression, risk factors, getting help, survivor support, and more / edited by Kim Wohlenhaus. -- 2nd ed.
    p. cm.
Includes bibliographical references and index.
    ISBN 978-0-7808-1088-4 (hbk. : alk. paper) 1. Teenagers--Suicidal behavior--Juvenile literature. 2. Suicidal behavior--Juvenile literature. 3. Suicide--Prevention--Juvenile literature. I. Wohlenhaus, Kim.
    HV6546.S8345 2010
    362.280835--dc22
                                                        2010015720

Table of Contents

Part Three: Recognizing And Treating Suicidal Ideation

Part Four: When Someone You Know Dies From Suicide

Part Five: Preventing Suicide

Part Six: If You Need More Information

Preface

About This Book

Teens often face a host of stressors and confusing feelings as they grow through the adolescent years. The emotions associated with puberty, self-doubt, confusion about the future, family problems, and school pressures can sometimes seem overwhelming, and statistics indicate that as many as one in five high school students seriously considers suicide. But suicidal behavior is not a normal response to stress. Mental health professionals claim that most teen suicide victims have a mental health disorder, a history of substance abuse, or both. When suicide risks are acknowledged and warning signs are heeded, many teens in distress can learn that the feelings that led them to consider suicide are treatable and that there is hope for the future.

Suicide Information for Teens, Second Edition provides updated information about suicide risks, causes, and prevention. It discusses mental health disorders and life-threatening behaviors linked to suicide risk, including depression, bi-polar disorder, anxiety disorders, schizophrenia, substance abuse, and self-injury. It offers suggestions for recognizing suicide warning signs, and it explains the most commonly used treatments for suicidal ideation, including counseling and medications. A section on suicide loss addresses the complex grief experienced by those who are affected by a suicide death. The book concludes with a list of crisis hotlines and a directory of additional resources for further information.

How To Use This Book

This book is divided into parts and chapters. Parts focus on broad areas of interest; chapters are devoted to single topics within a part.

Part One: Suicide Facts And Statistics provides information about the occurrence of suicide among people of different age groups in the United States and around the world and among people of different ethnic backgrounds. It discusses concerns related to balancing U.S. citizens' rights under the second amendment with the efforts to limit access to firearms (the leading cause of suicide death), and it explains how the stigma associated with receiving mental health services can contribute to suicide risk by making people less likely to seek appropriate care.

Part Two: Mental Health Disorders And Life-Threatening Behaviors Linked To Suicide Risk discusses the types of mental illness that have the highest statistical links to suicide risk, including depression, bipolar disorder, anxiety disorders, and schizophrenia. Alcohol and drug abuse, which are second only to depression and other mood disorders as the most frequent risk factors for suicide, are also addressed, and several chapters offer facts about other related concerns, including abusive relationships, self-injury, and eating disorders.

Part Three: Recognizing And Treating Suicidal Ideation offers tips about identifying the warning signs that may precede a suicide attempt and the psychological and medical treatments that are available for dealing with suicidal thoughts. Information is also provided about recovering from a suicide attempt and planning for the future.

Part Four: When Someone You Know Dies From Suicide explains the facets of grief often experienced by people left behind after a suicide. It offers suggestions for working through the grieving process and for supporting others who are grieving.

Part Five: Preventing Suicide discusses important components of mental health and offers practical suggestions for helping someone who may be depressed or experiencing suicidal thoughts. It considers suicide as a preventable problem and identifies ways in which suicidal behaviors can be reduced.

Part Six: If You Need More Information includes a list of crisis hotlines and a directory of organizations able to provide more information about suicide, suicide prevention, and suicide risk factors. It concludes with a list of online and print resources for suicide survivors.

Bibliographic Note

This volume contains documents and excerpts from publications issued by the following government agencies: Centers for Disease Control and Prevention (CDC); National Center for Injury Prevention and Control; National Institute of Mental Health; National Institute on Drug Abuse; National Mental Health Information Center; Substance Abuse and Mental Health Services Administration; U.S. Department of Veterans Affairs; U.S. Food and Drug Administration (FDA); and the U.S. Department of Health and Human Services.

In addition, this volume contains copyrighted documents and articles produced by the following organizations, publications, and individuals: American Association for Marriage and Family Therapy; American Association of Suicidology; American Hospice Foundation; American Psychological Association; BereavedBySuicide.com; Canadian Mental Health Association; Children's Room; Guilford Publications; Helpguide.org (c/o Center for Healthy Aging); Hospice of the North Shore; Jason Foundation; Johns Hopkins Bloomberg School of Public Health; Michelle Linn-Gust; Massachusetts Medical Society; National Sleep Foundation; Nemours Foundation; *New England Journal of Medicine*; SAVE: Suicide Awareness Voices of Education; siblingsurvivors.com; Ginny Sparrow; Trevor Project; World Fellowship for Schizophrenia and Allied Disorders; World Health Organization; and World Psychiatry.

The photograph on the front cover is from aldomurillo/iStockphoto.

Full citation information is provided on the first page of each chapter. Every effort has been made to secure all necessary rights to reprint the copyrighted material. If any omissions have been made, please contact Omnigraphics to make corrections for future editions.

Acknowledgements

In addition to the organizations listed above, special thanks are due to Liz Collins, research and permissions coordinator; Cherry Edwards, permissions assistant; Karen Bellenir, managing editor, Zachary Klimecki, editorial assistant; and Elizabeth Bellenir, prepress technician.

About the *Teen Health Series*

At the request of librarians serving today's young adults, the *Teen Health Series* was developed as a specially focused set of volumes within Omnigraphics' *Health Reference Series*. Each volume deals comprehensively with a topic selected according to the needs and interests of people in middle school and high school.

Teens seeking preventive guidance, information about disease warning signs, medical statistics, and risk factors for health problems will find answers to their questions in the *Teen Health Series*. The *Series*, however, is not intended to serve as a tool for diagnosing illness, in prescribing treatments, or as a substitute for the physician/patient relationship. All people concerned about medical symptoms or the possibility of disease are encouraged to seek professional care from an appropriate health care provider.

If there is a topic you would like to see addressed in a future volume of the *Teen Health Series*, please write to:

Editor
Teen Health Series
Omnigraphics, Inc.
P.O. Box 31-1640
Detroit, MI 48231

A Note about Spelling and Style

Teen Health Series editors use *Stedman's Medical Dictionary* as an authority for questions related to the spelling of medical terms and the *Chicago Manual of Style* for questions related to grammatical structures, punctuation, and other editorial concerns. Consistent adherence is not always possible, however, because the individual volumes within the *Series* include many documents from a wide variety of different producers and copyright holders, and the editor's primary goal is to present material from each source as accurately as is possible following the terms specified by each document's producer. This sometimes means that information in different chapters or sections may follow other guidelines and alternate spelling authorities. For example, occasionally a copyright holder may require that eponymous terms be shown in possessive forms (Crohn's disease vs. Crohn disease) or that British spelling norms be retained (leukaemia vs. leukemia).

Locating Information within the *Teen Health Series*

The *Teen Health Series* contains a wealth of information about a wide variety of medical topics. As the *Series* continues to grow in size and scope, locating the precise information needed by a specific student may become more challenging. To address this concern, information about books within the *Teen Health Series* is included in *A Contents Guide to the Health Reference Series*. The *Contents Guide* presents an extensive list of more than 15,000 diseases, treatments, and other topics of general interest compiled from the Tables of Contents and major index headings from the books of the *Teen Health Series* and *Health Reference Series*. To access *A Contents Guide to the Health Reference Series*, visit www.healthreferenceseries.com.

Our Advisory Board

We would like to thank the following advisory board members for providing guidance to the development of this *Series*:

Dr. Lynda Baker, Associate Professor of Library and Information Science, Wayne State University, Detroit, MI

Nancy Bulgarelli, William Beaumont Hospital Library, Royal Oak, MI

Karen Imarisio, Bloomfield Township Public Library, Bloomfield Township, MI

Karen Morgan, Mardigian Library, University of Michigan-Dearborn, Dearborn, MI

Rosemary Orlando, St. Clair Shores Public Library, St. Clair Shores, MI

Medical Consultant

Medical consultation services are provided to the *Teen Health Series* editors by David A. Cooke, MD, FACP. Dr. Cooke is a graduate of Brandeis

University, and he received his M.D. degree from the University of Michigan. He completed residency training at the University of Wisconsin Hospital and Clinics. He is board-certified in internal medicine. Dr. Cooke currently works as part of the University of Michigan Health System and practices in Ann Arbor, MI. In his free time, he enjoys writing, science fiction, and spending time with his family.

Part One

Suicide Facts And Statistics

Chapter 1

Suicide In The United States

Suicide is a major, preventable public health problem. In 2006, it was the eleventh leading cause of death in the United States, accounting for 33,300 deaths.[1] The overall rate was 10.9 suicide deaths per 100,000 people.[1] An estimated 12 to 25 attempted suicides occur per every suicide death.[1]

Suicidal behavior is complex. Some risk factors vary with age, gender, or ethnic group and may occur in combination or change over time.

What are the risk factors for suicide?

Research shows that risk factors for suicide include the following:

- Depression and other mental disorders, or a substance-abuse disorder (often in combination with other mental disorders). More than 90 percent of people who die by suicide have these risk factors.[2]

- Prior suicide attempt

- Family history of mental disorder or substance abuse

- Family history of suicide

- Family violence, including physical or sexual abuse

- Firearms in the home,[3] the method used in more than half of suicides

- Incarceration

About This Chapter: Text in this chapter is from "Suicide in the U.S.: Statistics and Prevention," National Institute of Mental Health, 2009.

- Exposure to the suicidal behavior of others, such as family members, peers, or media figures[2]

However, suicide and suicidal behavior are not normal responses to stress; many people have these risk factors, but are not suicidal. Research also shows that the risk for suicide is associated with changes in brain chemicals called neurotransmitters, including serotonin. Decreased levels of serotonin have been found in people with depression, impulsive disorders, and a history of suicide attempts, and in the brains of suicide victims.[4]

Are women or men at higher risk?

- Suicide was the seventh leading cause of death for males and the sixteenth leading cause of death for females in 2006.[1]

- Almost four times as many males as females die by suicide.[1]

- Firearms, suffocation, and poison are by far the most common methods of suicide, overall. However, men and women differ in the method used, as shown below.[1]

    - Suicide by firearms: Males 56%; Females 31%

    - Suicide by suffocation: Males 23%; Females 19%

    - Suicide by poisoning: Males 13%; Females 40%

✤ **It's A Fact!!**
The National Violent Death Reporting System includes information on the presence of alcohol and other substances at the time of death. For those tested for substances, the findings from 16 states revealed that one-third of those who died by suicide were positive for alcohol at the time of death and nearly one in five had evidence of opiates, including heroin and prescription pain killers.

Source: Excerpted from "Suicide: Facts at a Glance," National Center for Injury Prevention and Control, Centers for Disease Control and Prevention (CDC), Summer 2009.

Is suicide common among children and young people?

In 2006, suicide was the third leading cause of death for young people ages 15 to 24.[1] Of every 100,000 young people in each age group, the following number died by suicide:[1]

- Children ages 10 to 14: 1.3 per 100,000

- Adolescents ages 15 to 19: 8.2 per 100,000

- Young adults ages 20 to 24: 12.5 per 100,000

As in the general population, young people were much more likely to use firearms, suffocation, and poisoning than other methods of suicide, overall. However, while adolescents and young adults were more likely to use firearms than suffocation, children were dramatically more likely to use suffocation.[1]

There were also gender differences in suicide among young people, as follows:

- Over four times as many males as females ages 15 to 19 died by suicide.[1]

- More than six times as many males as females ages 20 to 24 died by suicide.[1]

Are older adults at risk?

Older Americans are disproportionately likely to die by suicide.

- Of every 100,000 people ages 65 and older, 14.2 died by suicide in 2006. This figure is higher than the national average of 10.9 suicides per 100,000 people in the general population.[1]

- Non-Hispanic white men age 85 or older had an even higher rate, with 48 suicide deaths per 100,000.[1]

Are some ethnic groups or races at higher risk?

Of every 100,000 people in each of the following ethnic/racial groups below, the following number died by suicide in 2006.[1]

- Highest rates:

  - American Indian and Alaska Natives—15.1 per 100,000

  - Non-Hispanic whites—13.9 per 100,000

- Lowest rates:

  - Hispanics—4.9 per 100,000

  - Non-Hispanic blacks—5.0 per 100,000

  - Asian and Pacific Islanders—5.7 per 100,000

❖ It's A Fact!!
**Largest Suicide Increase
Seen In Middle-Aged White Women**

The rate of suicide in the United States is increased for the first time in a decade, according to a new report from the Johns Hopkins Bloomberg School of Public Health's Center for Injury Research and Policy. The increase in the overall suicide rate between 1999 and 2005 was due primarily to an increase in suicides among whites aged 40–64, with white middle-aged women experiencing the largest annual increase. Whereas the overall suicide rate rose 0.7 percent during this time period, the rate among middle-aged white men rose 2.7 percent annually and 3.9 percent among middle-aged women. By contrast, suicide in blacks decreased significantly over the study's time period, and remained stable among Asian and Native Americans. The results are published online at the website of the *American Journal of Preventive Medicine* and will be published in the December [2008] print edition of the journal.

The researchers also conducted a detailed analysis of suicide methods across specific population groups. While firearms remain the predominant method, the rate of firearm suicides decreased during the study period. Suicide by poisoning increased markedly with a 6.3 percent annual increase among women, and a 2.3 percent annual increase among men. Hanging/suffocation accounted for 22 percent of all suicides by 2005, surpassing poisoning at 18 percent.

What are some risk factors for nonfatal suicide attempts?

As noted, an estimated 12 to 25 nonfatal suicide attempts occur per every suicide death. Men and the elderly are more likely to have fatal attempts than are women and youth.[1]

Risk factors for nonfatal suicide attempts by adults include depression and other mental disorders, alcohol and other substance abuse and separation or divorce.[5,6]

"The results underscore a change in the epidemiology of suicide, with middle-aged whites emerging as a new high-risk group," said study co-author Susan P. Baker, MPH, a professor with the Bloomberg School's Center for Injury Research and Policy. "Historically, suicide prevention programs have focused on groups considered to be at highest risk—teens and young adults of both genders as well as elderly white men. This research tells us we need to refocus our resources to develop prevention programs for men and women in their middle years."

Baker along with colleagues Guoqing Hu, PhD, Holly Wilcox, PhD, Lawrence Wissow, MD, MPH, analyzed data from the Web-based Injury Statistics Query and Reporting System (WISQARS) mortality reports, which provides data on deaths according to cause and intent of injury by age, race, gender and state. WISQARS mortality data are based on annual data files of the National Center for Health Statistics (NCHS) of the Centers for Disease Control and Prevention (CDC).

The reasons for the increase in the suicide rate are not fully understood. "While it would be straightforward to attribute the results to a rise in so-called mid-life crises, recent studies find that middle age is mostly a time of relative security and emotional well-being," said Baker. "Further research is warranted to explore societal changes that may be disproportionally affecting the middle-aged in this country."

Source: "U.S. Suicide Rate Increases," © 2008 Johns Hopkins Bloomberg School of Public Health (www.jhsph.edu). Reprinted with permission.

Risk factors for attempted suicide by youth include depression, alcohol or other drug-use disorder, physical or sexual abuse, and disruptive behavior.[6,7]

Most suicide attempts are expressions of extreme distress, not harmless bids for attention. A person who appears suicidal should not be left alone and needs immediate mental-health treatment.

What can be done to prevent suicide?

Research helps determine which factors can be modified to help prevent suicide and which interventions are appropriate for specific groups of people. Before being put into practice, prevention programs should be tested through research to determine their safety and effectiveness.[8] For example, because research has shown that mental and substance-abuse disorders are major risk factors for suicide, many programs also focus on treating these disorders as well as addressing suicide risk directly.

Studies showed that a type of psychotherapy called cognitive therapy reduced the rate of repeated suicide attempts by 50 percent during a year of follow-up. A previous suicide attempt is among the strongest predictors of subsequent suicide, and cognitive therapy helps suicide attempters consider alternative actions when thoughts of self-harm arise.[9]

Specific kinds of psychotherapy may be helpful for specific groups of people. For example, a treatment called dialectical behavior therapy reduced suicide attempts by half, compared with other kinds of therapy, in people with borderline personality disorder (a serious disorder of emotion regulation).[10]

The medication clozapine is approved by the Food and Drug Administration for suicide prevention in people with schizophrenia.[11] Other promising medications and psychosocial treatments for suicidal people are being tested.

Since research shows that older adults and women who die by suicide are likely to have seen a primary care provider in the year before death, improving primary-care providers' ability to recognize and treat risk factors may help prevent suicide among these groups.[12] Improving outreach to men at risk is a major challenge in need of investigation.

What should I do if I think someone is suicidal?

If you think someone is suicidal, do not leave him or her alone. Try to get the person to seek immediate help from his or her doctor or the nearest hospital emergency room, or call 911. Eliminate access to firearms or other potential tools for suicide, including unsupervised access to medications.

References

1. Centers for Disease Control and Prevention, National Center for Injury Prevention and Control. Web-based Injury Statistics Query and Reporting System (WISQARS): www.cdc.gov/ncipc/wisqars

2. Moscicki EK. Epidemiology of completed and attempted suicide: toward a framework for prevention. *Clinical Neuroscience Research*, 2001; 1: 310-23.

3. Miller M, Azrael D, Hepburn L, Hemenway D, Lippmann SJ. The association between changes in household firearm ownership and rates of suicide in the United States, 1981-2002. *Injury Prevention* 2006;12:178-182; doi:10.1136/ip.2005.010850.

4. Arango V, Huang YY, Underwood MD, Mann JJ. Genetics of the serotonergic system in suicidal behavior. *Journal of Psychiatric Research*. Vol. 37: 375-386. 2003.

5. Kessler RC, Borges G, Walters EE. Prevalence of and risk factors for lifetime suicide attempts in the National Comorbidity Survey. *Archives of General Psychiatry*, 1999; 56(7): 617-26.

6. Petronis KR, Samuels JF, Moscicki EK, Anthony JC. An epidemiologic investigation of potential risk factors for suicide attempts. *Social Psychiatry and Psychiatric Epidemiology*, 1990; 25(4): 193-9.

7. U.S. Public Health Service. National strategy for suicide prevention: goals and objectives for action. Rockville, MD: USDHHS, 2001.

8. Gould MS, Greenberg T, Velting DM, Shaffer D. Youth suicide risk and preventive interventions: a review of the past 10 years. *Journal of the American Academy of Child and Adolescent Psychiatry*, 2003; 42(4): 386-405.

9. Brown GK, Ten Have T, Henriques GR, Xie SX, Hollander JE, Beck AT. Cognitive therapy for the prevention of suicide attempts: a randomized controlled trial. *Journal of the American Medical Association* . 2005 Aug 3;294(5):563-70.

10. Linehan MM, Comtois KA, Murray AM, Brown MZ, Gallop RJ, Heard HL, Korslund KE, Tutek DA, Reynolds SK, Lindenboim N. Two-Year Randomized Controlled Trial and Follow-up of Dialectical Behavior Therapy vs Therapy by Experts for Suicidal Behaviors and Borderline Personality Disorder. *Archives of General Psychiatry*, 2006 Jul;63(7):757-766.

11. Meltzer HY, Alphs L, Green AI, Altamura AC, Anand R, Bertoldi A, Bourgeois M, Chouinard G, Islam MZ, Kane J, Krishnan R, Lindenmayer JP, Potkin S; International Suicide Prevention Trial Study Group. Clozapine treatment for suicidality in schizophrenia: International Suicide Prevention Trial (InterSePT). *Archives of General Psychiatry*, 2003; 60(1): 82-91.

12. Luoma JB, Pearson JL, Martin CE. Contact with mental health and primary care prior to suicide: a review of the evidence. *American Journal of Psychiatry*, 2002; 159: 909-16.

✔ **Quick Tip**

If you are in a crisis and need help right away, call this toll-free number, available 24 hours a day, every day: 1-800-273-TALK (8255). You will reach the National Suicide Prevention Lifeline, a service available to anyone. You may call for yourself or for someone you care about. All calls are confidential.

Source: National Institute of Mental Health, 2009.

Chapter 2

Statistics About Teen Suicide

Studying Suicide Trends Among Youths 10–24 Years Old

In 2004, suicide was the third leading cause of death among youths and young adults aged 10 to 24 years in the United States, accounting for 4,599 deaths. In the period between 1990 and 2003, the combined suicide rate for people 10–24 years old declined 28.5 percent, from 9.48 to 6.78 per 100,000 people. However, from 2003 to 2004, the rate increased by 8.0 percent, from 6.78 to 7.32, the largest single-year increase during 1990 to 2004.

To characterize U.S. trends in suicide among people aged 10–24 years old, the Centers for Disease Control and Prevention analyzed data recorded during the period of 1990 through 2004, the most recent data available. Results of that analysis indicated that, from 2003 to 2004, suicide rates for three sex-age groups (females 10–14 years old and 15–19 years old and males 15–19 years old) departed upward significantly from otherwise

About This Chapter: Text in this chapter is excerpted from "Suicide Trends Among Youths and Young Adults Aged 10–24 Years—United States, 1990–2004," reported by KM Lubell, PhD; SR Kegler, PhD; AE Crosby, MD; and D Karch, PhD, Division of Violence Prevention, National Center for Injury Prevention and Control, Centers for Disease Control and Prevention (CDC), *MMWR*, September 7, 2007, 56(35);905–908. The full text, including references and additional information about the statistical data, is available online at http://www.cdc.gov/mmwr/preview/mmwrhtml/mm5635a2.htm.

declining trends. Results further indicated that suicides both by hanging/ suffocation and poisoning among females 10–14 years old and 15–19 years old increased from 2003 to 2004 and were significantly in excess of trends in both groups.

In 1990, firearms were the most common suicide method among females in all three age groups examined, accounting for 55.2 percent of suicides in the group 10–14 years old, 56.0 percent in the group 15–19 years old, and 53.4 percent in the group 20–24 years old. However, from 1990 to 2004, among females in each of the three age groups, significant downward trends were observed in the rates both for firearm suicides and poisoning suicides, and a significant increase was observed in the rate for suicides by hanging/ suffocation. In 2004, hanging/suffocation was the most common method among females in all three age groups. Aside from 2004, the only other significant departure from trend among females in these two age groups during 1990 though 2004 was in suicides by hanging/suffocation among females 15–19 years old in 1996.

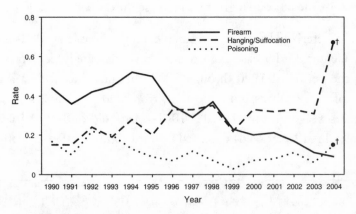

* Per 100,000 population.
† Standardized Pearson residual >2.

Figure 2.1. *Yearly suicide rates for females aged 10–14 years, by method—National Vital Statistics System, United States, 1990–2004.*

Table 2.1. Suicide rates* for youths and young adults aged 10–24 years, by age group, method, sex, and year — National Vital Statistics System, United States, 1990–2004

	10–14 yrs				15–19 yrs				20–24 yrs			
Sex/Year	All methods†	Firearm	Hanging/ Suffocation§	Poisoning¶	All methods	Firearm	Hanging/ Suffocation	Poisoning	All methods	Firearm	Hanging/ Suffocation	Poisoning
Females												
1990	0.80	0.44	0.15**	0.17**	3.73	2.09	0.55	0.89	4.11	2.19	0.43	1.15
1991	0.67	0.36	0.15**	0.10**	3.70	1.83	0.59	1.09	3.88	1.79	0.52	1.11
1992	0.90	0.42	0.24	0.22**	3.42	1.62	0.62	1.03	3.84	1.92	0.58	1.02
1993	0.93	0.45	0.19**	0.20**	3.80	2.00	0.62	0.92	4.36	2.11	0.59	1.24††
1994	0.95	0.52	0.28	0.13**	3.44	1.99	0.51	0.74	3.87	2.00	0.61	0.82
1995	0.82	0.50	0.20**	0.09**	3.07	1.64	0.57	0.62	4.21	2.15††	0.80	0.97
1996	0.80	0.35	0.33	0.07**	3.49	1.69	1.02††	0.51	3.57	1.65	0.71	0.88
1997	0.76	0.29	0.33	0.12**	3.31	1.70	0.95	0.47	3.59	1.63	0.88	0.75
1998	0.86	0.37	0.35	0.07**	2.84	1.43	0.81	0.38	3.70	1.72	0.87	0.65
1999	0.51	0.23	0.22	0.03**	2.75	1.11	0.89	0.48	3.37	1.36	0.84	0.79
2000	0.62	0.20**	0.33	0.07**	2.75	1.06	1.02	0.42	3.23	1.29	0.78	0.70
2001	0.64	0.21	0.32	0.08**	2.70	0.96	0.99	0.52	3.06	1.03	0.87	0.83
2002	0.62	0.17**	0.33	0.11**	2.36	0.75	0.98	0.43	3.48	1.18	0.95	0.92
2003	0.54	0.11**	0.31	0.06**	2.66	0.77	1.24	0.43	3.39	1.18	1.10	0.82
2004	0.95††	0.09**	0.68††	0.15**††	3.52††	0.98	1.72††	0.54††	3.59	1.14	1.23	0.76
Males												
1990	2.17	1.19§§	0.91	0.02**	18.17	12.63§§	3.48††	1.49	25.69	16.69§§	5.19	2.41
1991	2.28	1.37	0.78	0.08**	17.92	12.70	3.16	1.26	25.40	16.97	4.52	2.51
1992	2.40	1.44	0.80	0.11**	17.61	12.59	3.17	1.20	25.42	16.79	5.04	2.11
1993	2.40	1.51	0.78	0.04**	17.39	12.29	3.20	1.11	26.47	18.04	4.94	2.23
1994	2.36	1.43	0.79	0.08**	17.95††	13.11††	3.27	0.74	27.96††	18.80††	5.21	2.30
1995	2.57	1.38	1.06	0.06**	17.11	11.86	3.39	0.85	27.01††	17.27	5.96††	1.96
1996	2.23	1.29	0.90	0.01**	15.38	10.20	3.50	0.88	24.47	15.73	5.36	1.79
1997	2.29	0.98	1.21	0.03**	14.94	9.78	3.84	0.51§§	22.66	14.34	5.02	1.79
1998	2.30	1.15	1.12	0.01**	14.34	9.31	3.57	0.65	22.33	13.71	5.72	1.50
1999	1.85	0.77	0.99	0.03**	13.05	8.40	3.36§§	0.54	20.85	12.81	4.80§§	1.61
2000	2.26	0.86	1.28	0.08**††	13.00	7.63	3.98	0.67	21.40	12.90	5.66	1.32
2001	1.93	0.64	1.21	0.02**	12.87	7.11	4.33	0.63	20.37	11.76	5.92	1.38
2002	1.81	0.63	1.11	0.00**	12.22	6.38	4.32	0.72	20.62	11.78	6.11	1.11
2003	1.73	0.57	1.11	0.03**	11.61	6.26	4.22	0.57	20.21	11.42	6.26	1.16
2004	1.71	0.46	1.24	0.00**	12.65††	6.47	4.71	0.66	20.84	11.12	6.63	1.49††

* Per 100,000 population in sex-age group.
† Includes cutting, jumping, burning, drowning, and other or unspecified methods.
§ Includes self-inflicted asphyxiation and ligature strangulation.
¶ Includes intentional drug overdose and carbon monoxide exposure.
** Unstable rate based on 20 or fewer deaths.
†† Standardized Pearson residual >2.
§§ Standardized Pearson residual <-2.

Figure 2.1. *Yearly suicide rates for females aged 10–14 years, by method—National Vital Statistics System, United States, 1990–2004.*

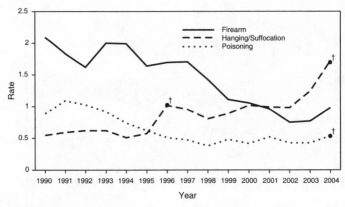

*Per 100,000 population.
†Standardized Pearson residual >2.

Figure 2.2. *Yearly suicide rates for females aged 15–19 years, by method—National Vital Statistics System, United States, 1990–2004.*

Discussion Of Findings

The findings in this report indicate that 2004 suicide rates for males 15–19 years old and females 10–14 years old and 15–19 years old diverged upward significantly from modeled trends during 1990 through 2004. For females in the two age groups, significant departures were observed for 2004 in suicides by hanging/suffocation and poisoning. The rate for suicide by hanging/suffocation among females 10–14 years old more than doubled from 2003 to 2004, from 0.31 to 0.68 per 100,000 of the population. During the period of 1990 through 2003, the highest yearly rate for such deaths among females in this age group was 0.35 per 100,000 of the population in 1998.

❖ **It's A Fact!!**
One comparative study, conducted in Singapore, suggested that perceptions of interpersonal relationship problems are more common among young female suicide decedents than among their male counterparts. Family discord, legal/disciplinary problems, school concerns, and mental health conditions such as depression increase the risk for suicide among youths of both sexes. Drug/alcohol use can exacerbate these problems.

> ### 🖙 Remember!!
>
> These findings demonstrate the potential mutability of youth suicidal behavior. Public health researchers and suicide-prevention practitioners need to learn more about both the risk factors for suicide among young females and effective strategies for suicide prevention. The trends in suicide rates and methods described in this report, if confirmed, suggest that prevention measures focused solely on restricting access to the most lethal means are likely to have limited success. Prevention measures should address the underlying reasons for suicide in populations that are vulnerable.

The marked increases in suicide rates among females in the two younger age groups suggest possible changes in risk factors for suicide and the methods used, with greater use of methods that are readily accessible.

Scientific knowledge regarding risk factors for suicide in young females is limited. Research that focuses on suicide mortality has emphasized males, who constitute approximately three fourths of suicide decedents 10–19 years old. In contrast, research on suicidal behavior among females primarily has examined factors related to suicidal thoughts and nonfatal self-inflicted injuries.

Recent reports have detailed unintentional asphyxia fatalities resulting from adolescents playing "the choking game" (that is, intentionally restricting the supply of oxygen to the brain, often with a ligature, to induce a brief euphoria). Some of these fatalities likely are misclassified as suicides. However, such deaths are unlikely to account for a substantial portion of the recent increases in hanging/suffocation suicides among young girls. The available evidence suggests that choking-game fatalities occur predominantly among boys. In addition, analysis of hanging/suffocation deaths classified as unintentional or undetermined in this population did not reveal increases that paralleled those in hanging/suffocation suicides.

The findings in this report are subject to at least three limitations. First, because U.S. mortality data currently are available only through 2004, whether the increases observed in 2004 represent changes in trends or single-year anomalies is not clear and suggests a need for further study as more current data become available. Second, official mortality data for suicides might include classification errors. Previous research has highlighted the extent to which suicides are undercounted. Finally, because U.S. mortality data include limited variables, these data do not allow examination of potential differences or changes in the underlying risk factors for fatal suicidal behavior among young females. Other data sources (for example, the National Violent Death Reporting System) that collect a broader array of information about the circumstances surrounding suicides might provide additional insights.

Chapter 3

Teen Suicide: A Global Perspective

Abstract

Global suicide rates among adolescents in the 15–19 age group, according to the latest World Health Organization (WHO) Mortality Database, were examined. Data for this age group were available from 90 countries (in some cases areas) out of the 130 WHO member states. The mean suicide rate for this age group, based on data available for the latest year, was 7.4/100,000. Suicide rates were higher in males (10.5) than in females (4.1). This applies in almost all countries. The exceptions are China, Cuba, Ecuador, El Salvador, and Sri Lanka, where the female suicide rate was higher than the male. In the 90 countries (areas) studied, suicide was the fourth leading cause of death among young males and the third for young females. Of the 132,423 deaths of young people in the 90 countries, suicide accounted for 9.1%. The trend of suicide rates from 26 countries (areas) with data available during the period 1965–1999 was also studied. A rising trend of suicide in young males was observed. This was particularly marked in the years before 1980 and in countries outside Europe. The WHO database is the largest of its kind and, indeed, the only information source that can currently be used for analysis of global mortality due to suicide. Methodological limitations are discussed.

About This Chapter: "Global suicide rates among young people aged 15–19," by Danuta Wasserman, Qi Cheng, and Guo-xin Jiang. *World Psychiatry*, 4;2. 114–120, June 2005. The complete text of this article is available at http://www.ncbi.nlm.nih.gov/pmc/articles/ PMC1414751/. This article has been corrected. See *World Psychiatry*. 2006 February; 5(1): 39. © Copyright 2006 World Psychiatric Association. Reprinted with permission.

Introduction

Suicidal behavior is a major health concern in many countries, developed and developing alike. At least a million people are estimated to die annually from suicide worldwide (1). Many more people, especially the young and middle-aged, attempt suicide (2). Over the last few decades, while suicide rates have been reported as stable or falling in many developed countries, a rising trend of youth suicide has been observed. In 21 of the 30 countries in the World Health Organization (WHO) European region, suicide rates in males aged 15–19 rose between 1979 and 1996. For females, suicide rates rose less markedly in 18 of the 30 countries studied (3). Various possible explanations for these rising suicide trends—loss of social cohesion, breakdown of traditional family structure, growing economic instability and unemployment, and rising prevalence of depressive disorders—have been presented.

Some worldwide analyses of suicide trends and rates in the world have been published (4–7), but very little is known worldwide about the causes of death and suicide rates among young people aged 15–19.

The purpose of this study was to present an overall picture of suicide among adolescents worldwide using available data from the WHO database, and to evaluate the role of suicide as a cause of death in the 15–19 age group.

Methods

Data on causes of death and population for each country (area) were downloaded from the WHO Mortality Database website in February 2004. Statistics on causes of death and population in the 15–19 age group were available for 90 countries (areas) in the year 1980 or later. From 71% of these 90 countries (areas), there were data relating to the year 1995 or later, and roughly half had data for 2000 or later. For 30%, there were figures dating back to before 1995.

The downloaded data files were converted into SPSS files [a type of computer file for statistical information]. Data files with different versions of the International Classification of Diseases (ICD) were merged and analyzed by gender, age group, cause of death, and calendar year.

The following codes for certain suicide in the WHO Mortality Database were used: in ICD-7 classification, codes A148 and B049, including E963, E970-E979; in ICD-8 classification, codes A147 and B049, including E950-E959; in ICD-9 classification, codes B54 and C102, including E950-E959; in ICD-10 classification, codes X60-X84 (in some countries code 1101, including codes X60-X84).

The mean suicide rate in the 15–19 age group was calculated by collating the numbers of suicides in the latest year with available figures in the population from all the 90 countries (areas). Moreover, to avoid confounding country effects with time effects, only countries that reported data for the same year were selected. Therefore, suicide rates in 63 countries in 1995 were also analyzed and compared, since the largest number of countries (areas) reported suicide and population data for that year.

A few countries were excluded from the analyses since the population in the 15–19 age group numbered less than 10,000.

In order to evaluate suicide trends, suicide rates from all countries (areas) with data available throughout the period 1965–1999 were examined. Rates in European and non-European countries were compared.

The total number of deaths for the 90 countries (areas) with the latest available data was divided by the number of deaths in each diagnostic category to arrive at percentages for causes of death in each category. The "other causes of death" category includes many different causes that account for relatively small numbers of deaths, such as diseases of the blood and blood-forming organs; diseases of the eye, ear, skin and subcutaneous tissue, musculoskeletal system and connective tissue, and genitourinary system; certain conditions originating in the perinatal period; and various symptoms, signs and ill-defined conditions.

Results

For 90 countries (areas), data were available both on causes of death and on the population aged 15-19. The numbers of suicides and rates per 100,000 persons aged 15–19 and the latest year in which data were available for each country (area) are presented in Table 3.1.

Table 3.1. Suicide numbers and rates per 100,000 young persons aged 15–19 in 90 countries (areas), according to the WHO Mortality Database, February 2004 (latest available data for each country or area).

Country (area)	Year	Number			Rate		
		Males	Females	Total	Males	Females	Total
Sri Lanka	1986	388	424	812	43.9	49.3	46.5
Lithuania	2002	54	12	66	38.4	8.8	23.9
Russian Federation	2002	2,384	499	2,883	38.5	8.3	23.6
Kazakhstan	2002	240	78	318	31.2	10.5	21.0
Luxembourg	2002	3	1	4	23.5	8.2	16.0
New Zealand	2000	31	11	42	22.3	8.2	15.3
El Salvador	1993	44	52	96	13.2	15.8	14.5
Belarus	2001	100	16	116	23.6	3.9	14.0
Estonia	2002	13	1	14	24.1	1.9	13.2
Turkmenistan	1998	41	21	62	16.6	8.8	12.8
Ukraine	2000	375	92	467	19.6	4.9	12.4
Ireland	2000	34	7	41	19.8	4.3	12.3
Mauritius	2000	5	6	11	10.1	12.5	11.3
Norway	2001	21	8	29	15.3	6.2	10.9
Canada	2000	173	52	225	16.3	5.2	10.8
Latvia	2002	16	4	20	16.9	4.4	10.8
Kyrgyzstan	2002	42	13	55	15.2	4.8	10.0
Virgin Islands (USA)	1980	1	0	1	20.0	0.0	9.8
Barbados	1995	1	1	2	9.6	9.8	9.7
Austria	2002	37	9	46	15.1	3.8	9.6
Trinidad and Tobago	1994	6	6	12	8.9	10.5	9.6
Finland	2002	25	6	31	15.0	3.8	9.5
Uzbekistan	2000	170	86	256	12.5	6.4	9.5
Belgium	1997	46	12	58	14.5	3.9	9.3
Cuba	1996	23	45	68	6.1	12.5	9.2
Ecuador	1991	40	64	104	6.9	11.4	9.1
Iceland	1999	1	1	2	9.0	9.3	9.1
Australia	2001	95	25	120	13.8	3.8	8.9
Singapore	2001	10	8	18	9.2	7.8	8.5
Suriname	1990	3	1	4	12.5	4.3	8.5
Poland	2001	242	39	281	14.1	2.4	8.4
Switzerland	2000	27	8	35	12.6	4.0	8.4
Croatia	2002	21	3	24	14.0	2.1	8.2

Table 3.1. Continued

Country (area)	Year	Number			Rate		
		Males	Females	Total	Males	Females	Total
USA	2000	1,347	269	1,616	13.0	2.7	8.0
Grenada	1988	0	1	1	0.0	15.6	7.8
Slovenia	1987	8	2	10	12.0	3.1	7.6
Hungary	2002	37	12	49	11.2	3.8	7.5
Guadeloupe	1981	2	1	3	8.8	4.6	6.8
Japan	2000	335	138	473	8.8	3.8	6.4
Uruguay	1990	11	5	16	8.3	3.9	6.2
Bulgaria	2002	25	6	31	9.2	2.3	5.8
Czech Republic	2001	33	6	39	9.5	1.8	5.7
Argentina	1996	122	67	189	7.1	4.0	5.6
Costa Rica	1995	13	7	20	7.1	4.0	5.6
Germany	2001	207	54	261	8.7	2.4	5.6
Thailand	1994	189	154	343	6.1	5.1	5.6
Colombia	1994	120	73	193	6.7	4.2	5.5
Venezuela	1994	80	41	121	7.1	3.8	5.5
Republic of Korea	2001	110	85	195	5.9	4.9	5.4
Hong Kong	1999	12	12	24	5.1	5.3	5.2
France	1999	150	48	198	7.5	2.5	5.0
Denmark	1999	13	1	14	9.0	0.7	4.9
Israel	1999	24	2	26	8.7	0.8	4.9
Paraguay (reporting areas)	1987	5	7	12	3.9	5.6	4.7
Romania	2002	59	18	77	7.0	2.2	4.7
Netherlands	2000	35	8	43	7.4	1.8	4.6
Sweden	2001	15	7	22	5.7	2.8	4.3
Brazil (South, South-East and Central West)	1995	286	128	414	5.7	2.6	4.2
Puerto Rico	1992	14	0	14	8.3	0.0	4.2
United Kingdom	1999	122	33	155	6.5	1.8	4.2
Republic of Moldova	2002	13	2	15	7.1	1.1	4.1
China (selected rural and urban areas)	1999	179	253	432	3.2	4.8	4.0
Belize	1995	0	1	1	0.0	7.9	3.9

Table 3.1. Continued

Country (area)	Year	Number			Rate		
		Males	Females	Total	Males	Females	Total
Slovakia	2002	13	4	17	5.8	1.9	3.9
Chile	1994	38	8	46	6.2	1.3	3.8
Mexico	1995	263	117	380	5.1	2.3	3.7
Spain	2000	71	18	89	5.3	1.4	3.4
Panama	1987	6	2	8	4.6	1.6	3.1
Albania	2001	4	5	9	2.8	3.3	3.0
Dominican Republic	1985	10	12	22	2.7	3.2	2.9
Italy	2000	57	25	82	3.6	1.7	2.7
Macedonia	2000	1	3	4	1.2	3.7	2.4
Tajikistan	1999	11	3	14	3.3	0.9	2.1
Portugal	2000	9	3	12	2.6	0.9	1.8
Greece	1999	10	2	12	2.7	0.6	1.7
Guyana	1984	2	0	2	3.4	0.0	1.7
Armenia	2002	2	1	3	1.3	0.6	1.0
Peru	1983	13	7	20	1.3	0.7	1.0
Jamaica	1985	2	0	2	1.4	0.0	0.7
Azerbaijan	2002	5	0	5	1.1	0.0	0.6
Syrian Arab Republic (part)	1985	5	0	5	1.0	0.0	0.5
Georgia	2000	1	0	1	0.6	0.0	0.3
Egypt	1987	0	1	1	0.0	0.04	0.02
Bahamas	1995	0	0	0	0.0	0.0	0.0
Guatemala	1984	0	0	0	0.0	0.0	0.0
Kuwait	2001	0	0	0	0.0	0.0	0.0
Malta	2002	0	0	0	0.0	0.0	0.0
Philippines	1996	0	0	0	0.0	0.0	0.0
Saint Lucia	1988	0	0	0	0.0	0.0	0.0
Saint Vincent and Grenadines	1986	0	0	0	0.0	0.0	0.0
Total		8,801	3,263	12,064	10.5	4.1	7.4

Source: *World Psychiatry*. 2005 June; 4(2): 114–120.

A total of 12,064 cases of suicide (8,801 males and 3,263 females) from 90 countries (areas) were analyzed. The mean suicide rate for 15–19 year-olds in the 90 countries (areas), based on data in different years for the various countries, was 7.4/100,000 (10.5 for males and 4.1 for females).

There were 13 countries with suicide rates 1.5 times or more above the mean: these included Sri Lanka, with the highest suicide rate, followed by Lithuania, Russia, and Kazakhstan. In 24 countries (areas) suicide rates were above, but less than 1.5 times, the mean: this category included Norway, Canada, Latvia, Austria, Finland, Belgium, and the USA. The remaining 53 countries (areas) had below-average suicide rates (Table 3.1).

The mean suicide rate for males and females together in the 63 countries (areas) for which data for the year 1995 were available was 8.4/100,000, slightly higher than that (7.4/100,000) in the 90 countries (areas) described above, mainly owing to the higher suicide rate in males (Table 3.2). Among these, 13 countries (including Russia, New Zealand, the Baltic states, Kazakhstan, Norway, Canada, and Slovenia) reported suicide rates of 1.5 times the mean or more. Sixteen countries (including Ukraine, Switzerland, the USA, Austria, Ireland, Belgium, Hungary, and Portugal) showed suicide rates above, but less than 1.5 times, the mean. Thirty-four countries had below-average suicide rates (Table 3.2). More than two-thirds of the countries listed in Table 3.2 are European countries.

In 26 countries (areas), data were available for the whole period studied, 1965–1999. Table 3.3 presents suicide rates for each country (area), broken down by gender, during three periods (1965–1979, 1980–1989 and 1990–1999). A rising trend of suicide rates in the 15–19 age group was observed in males from both non-European and European countries, while the trend was fairly stable or declined slightly in females. Suicide rates among both young males and females were higher in non-European than in European countries during the whole period 1965–1999 (Table 3.3).

Causes of death were examined for 90 countries (areas). The data covered the same years as the data presented in Table 3.1. A total of 132,423 deaths from all kinds of causes in the 15–19 age group in the 90 countries (areas) (Table 3.4) were analyzed. The most common cause of death for both males

Table 3.2. Suicide numbers and rates per 100,000 young persons aged 15–19 in the 63 countries (areas) for which data are available for the year 1995.

Country (area)	Number			Rate		
	Males	Females	Total	Males	Females	Total
Russian Federation	1,988	509	2,497	36.5	9.6	23.2
New Zealand	45	14	59	33.0	10.6	22.0
Lithuania	42	8	50	32.7	6.4	19.7
Kazakhstan	222	69	291	29.3	9.2	19.3
Latvia	21	5	26	25.1	6.1	15.7
Estonia	12	3	15	23.6	6.2	15.1
Finland	42	6	48	25.1	3.7	14.7
Belarus	89	16	105	23.7	4.3	14.0
Kyrgyzstan	36	26	62	16.1	11.8	14.0
Norway	28	8	36	20.3	6.1	13.4
Canada	217	47	264	21.4	4.9	13.3
Cuba	41	58	99	10.5	15.5	12.9
Slovenia	15	4	19	19.3	5.5	12.6
Mauritius	8	5	13	14.7	9.4	12.1
Ukraine	334	93	427	18.1	5.2	11.7
Switzerland	32	14	46	15.7	7.2	11.6
Czech Republic	72	19	91	16.2	4.5	10.5
USA	1,616	274	1,89	17.4	3.1	10.5
Austria	44	3	47	18.6	1.3	10.2
Ireland	29	5	34	16.9	3.1	10.1
Barbados	1	1	2	9.6	9.8	9.7
Iceland	2	0	2	18.7	0.0	9.5
Bulgaria	43	15	58	13.4	4.9	9.3
Australia	87	27	114	13.4	4.4	9.0
Luxembourg	1	1	2	8.8	9.2	9.0
Belgium	38	17	55	12.1	5.6	8.9
Hungary	65	9	74	15.3	2.2	8.9
Croatia	24	5	29	14.2	3.1	8.8
Poland	234	46	280	14.2	2.9	8.7
Republic of Moldova	21	8	29	11.4	4.4	7.9
Republic of Korea	181	108	289	8.9	5.6	7.3
Sweden	27	9	36	10.3	3.6	7.1
Turkmenistan	27	4	32	12.1	1.8	7.0

Table 3.2. Continued

Country (area)	Number			Rate		
	Males	Females	Total	Males	Females	Total
China (selected rural and urban areas)	227	373	600	4.9	8.7	6.7
Slovakia	27	5	32	11.1	2.1	6.7
Germany	220	66	286	9.9	3.1	6.6
Singapore	8	5	13	7.7	5.2	6.5
Israel	22	9	31	8.5	3.7	6.1
Costa Rica	13	7	20	7.1	4.0	5.6
Denmark	15	2	17	9.1	1.3	5.3
France	151	51	202	7.7	2.7	5.3
Romania	78	26	104	7.8	2.7	5.3
Uzbekistan	89	34	123	7.6	3.0	5.3
Argentina	113	60	173	6.7	3.6	5.2
Japan	287	136	423	6.6	3.3	5.0
Hong Kong	14	6	20	6.4	3.0	4.7
Brazil (South, South-East and Central West)	286	128	414	5.7	2.6	4.2
United Kingdom	106	31	137	6.0	1.8	4.0
Belize	0	1	1	0.0	7.9	3.9
Spain	100	21	121	6.2	1.4	3.9
Mexico	263	117	380	5.1	2.3	3.7
Tajikistan	15	6	21	5.2	2.1	3.6
Malta	1	0	1	6.8	0.0	3.5
Netherlands	21	11	32	4.4	2.4	3.5
Albania	5	4	9	3.7	2.7	3.2
Italy	81	22	103	4.4	1.2	2.9
Portugal	15	8	23	3.7	2.0	2.9
Greece	9	6	15	2.3	1.6	2.0
Macedonia	1	1	2	1.2	1.2	1.2
Armenia	2	1	3	1.2	0.6	0.9
Kuwait	1	0	1	1.7	0.0	0.9
Azerbaijan	4	0	4	1.2	0.0	0.6
Bahamas	0	0	0	0.0	0.0	0.0
Total	7,859	2,573	10,432	12.4	4.2	8.4

Source: *World Psychiatry*. 2005 June; 4(2): 114–120.

Table 3.3. Suicide rates per 100,000 young persons aged 15–19 in 26 countries (areas) with data available for 1965–1999

	Males			Females			Total		
	1965-79	1980-89	1990-99	1965-79	1980-89	1990-99	1965-79	1980-89	1990-99
Mauritius	5.08	6.16	11.69	9.02	11.06	13.17	7.04	8.58	12.42
Canada	13.75	20.74	19.85	3.38	3.65	4.95	8.66	12.40	12.59
USA	10.22	15.30	16.48	2.84	3.66	3.38	6.57	9.59	10.11
Hong Kong	3.01	3.38	5.87	4.65	3.63	4.95	3.81	3.50	5.43
Japan	10.61	7.46	6.60	6.91	3.99	3.24	8.79	5.77	4.96
Singapore	4.99	5.19	6.33	7.48	7.42	4.37	6.20	6.27	5.38
Australia	9.12	14.13	16.89	3.50	3.05	4.15	6.37	8.72	10.68
New Zealand	7.49	17.51	28.60	2.96	4.24	9.80	5.28	11.01	19.33
Non-European countries	10.34	13.17	13.83	4.08	3.78	3.59	7.25	8.58	8.84
Austria	16.67	19.43	16.70	5.26	6.60	3.68	11.08	13.13	10.36
Bulgaria	7.55	10.22	12.20	5.15	5.89	4.25	6.38	8.11	8.32
Denmark	6.14	9.18	8.02	2.99	3.31	2.43	4.61	6.32	5.29
Finland	18.94	24.54	25.90	4.99	5.25	4.65	12.12	15.09	15.51
France	6.54	7.95	7.62	3.25	2.85	2.80	4.92	5.46	5.26
Greece	1.51	2.61	2.17	1.72	1.72	0.76	1.61	2.18	1.49
Hungary	19.59	16.23	13.81	8.01	6.82	3.94	13.92	11.67	9.00
Iceland	9.97	20.91	26.72	0.66	0.00	6.71	5.45	10.67	16.91
Ireland	2.57	6.80	14.96	0.68	1.12	3.09	1.65	4.03	9.17
Italy	2.52	2.93	4.23	1.87	1.05	1.35	2.20	2.01	2.82
Luxembourg	9.24	12.00	13.04	3.20	6.24	4.57	6.28	9.18	8.91
Netherlands	3.78	4.09	5.62	1.22	1.76	2.37	2.53	2.95	4.03
Norway	7.04	15.71	17.37	1.92	3.45	6.63	4.54	9.74	12.12
Portugal	4.83	5.30	2.88	3.77	4.62	1.68	4.30	4.96	2.29
Spain	1.89	4.03	4.85	0.79	1.16	1.43	1.35	2.63	3.18
Sweden	8.69	8.46	8.27	5.48	3.84	4.23	7.12	6.21	6.30
Switzerland	14.87	18.63	13.64	5.35	4.58	4.29	10.16	11.77	9.09
United Kingdom	3.49	4.95	5.92	1.84	1.42	1.65	2.68	3.23	3.85
European countries	5.50	6.61	7.13	2.67	2.35	2.26	4.11	4.53	4.75
All countries	9.12	11.41	12.14	3.73	3.40	3.26	6.46	7.49	7.82

Source: *World Psychiatry*. 2005 June; 4(2): 114–120.

and females was "transport accidents," which accounted for approximately one-fifth of deaths. Suicide ranked fourth as a cause of death for males, and third for females. Suicide accounted for 9.1% of all deaths among male and female adolescents together: 9.5% and 8.2% respectively (Table 3.4).

A similar rank order of different categories of causes of death was also seen from the analysis of mortality data for the 63 countries (areas) from which data were available for the same year, that is, 1995 (data not shown).

Table 3.4. Causes of death for young persons aged 15-19 in 90 countries (areas), according to the WHO Mortality Database, February 2004 (latest available data for each country or area)

Causes of death	Male		Female		Total	
	N	%	N	%	N	%
Transport accidents	19,643	21.2	6,919	17.4	26,562	20.1
Other accidents	19,274	20.8	5,084	12.8	24,358	18.4
Assault	13,735	14.8	2,108	5.3	15,843	12.0
Suicide	8,801	9.5	3,263	8.2	12,064	9.1
Neoplasms	5,017	5.4	3,585	9.0	8,602	6.5
Diseases of the circulatory system	4,966	5.4	3,484	8.8	8,450	6.4
Diseases of the nervous system	3,765	4.1	2,230	5.6	5,995	4.5
Diseases of the respiratory system	2,878	3.1	2,061	5.2	4,939	3.7
Infective and parasitic diseases	2,580	2.8	2,116	5.3	4,696	3.5
Diseases of the digestive system	1,420	1.5	940	2.4	2,360	1.8
Congenital malformations, deformations	1,061	1.1	817	2.1	1,878	1.4
Endocrine, nutritional and metabolic diseases	850	0.9	859	2.2	1,709	1.3
Mental and behavioral disorders	457	0.5	188	0.5	645	0.5
Other causes	8,296	8.9	6,026	15.2	14,322	10.8
Total	92,743	100.0	39,680	100.0	132,423	100.0

Source: *World Psychiatry.* 2005 June; 4(2): 114–120.

✦ It's A Fact!!

Suicide Prevention
The Problem

- Every year, almost one million people die from suicide; a "global" mortality rate of 16 per 100,000, or one death every 40 seconds.

- In the last 45 years suicide rates have increased by 60% worldwide. Suicide is among the three leading causes of death among those aged 15–44 years in some countries, and the second leading cause of death in the 10–24 years age group; these figures do not include suicide attempts which are up to 20 times more frequent than completed suicide.

- Suicide worldwide is estimated to represent 1.8% of the total global burden of disease in 1998, and 2.4% in countries with market and former socialist economies in 2020.

- Although traditionally suicide rates have been highest among the male elderly, rates among young people have been increasing to such an extent that they are now the group at highest risk in a third of countries, in both developed and developing countries.

- Mental disorders (particularly depression and alcohol use disorders) are a major risk factor for suicide in Europe and North America; however, in Asian countries impulsiveness plays an important role. Suicide is complex with psychological, social, biological, cultural and environmental factors involved.

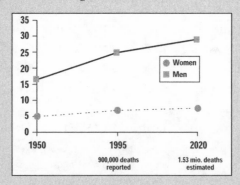

Figure 3.1. *Reported (1950–1995) and estimated (2020) suicide rates in reporting countries.*

Effective Interventions

- Strategies involving restriction of access to common methods of suicide, such as firearms or toxic substances like pesticides, have proved to be effective in reducing suicide rates; however, there is a need to adopt multisectoral approaches involving many levels of intervention and activities.

- There is compelling evidence indicating that adequate prevention and treatment of depression and alcohol and substance abuse can reduce suicide rates, as well as follow-up contact with those who have attempted suicide.

Challenges And Obstacles

- Worldwide, the prevention of suicide has not been adequately addressed due to basically a lack of awareness of suicide as a major problem and the taboo in many societies to discuss openly about it. In fact, only a few countries have included prevention of suicide among their priorities.

- Reliability of suicide certification and reporting is an issue in great need of improvement.

It is clear that suicide prevention requires intervention also from outside the health sector and calls for an innovative, comprehensive multisectoral approach, including both health and non-health sectors, for example, education, labour, police, justice, religion, law, politics, the media.

Suicide rates varied substantially among the countries, by a factor of up to 100. However, it must been borne in mind that some countries have small populations and that there can be major random variations in the annual number of suicides. Although the data presented here are an acceptable basis for evaluating the global impact of suicide on young people, it should be kept in mind that relevant data are still lacking from a number of countries. For a more definitive and correct view of suicide worldwide, data collection from these countries is needed.

Discussion

Suicide data are still not available in many countries. In the present study, data from only 90 countries (areas) out of the world's 192 nations were available for the 15–19 age group in the WHO Mortality Database, which is the largest database in the world on this topic. The WHO mortality statistics are commonly broken down by gender and age. However, some countries do not report deaths broken down for the 15–19 age group, and there are only 130 member states of WHO.

The reliability of suicide statistics is often questioned (4). Suicides are underreported for cultural and religious reasons, as well as owing to different classification and ascertainment procedures. Suicide can be masked by many other diagnostic categories of causes of death. Unfortunately, in cases of young people, death due to suicide is often misclassified or masked by other mortality diagnoses. This makes the global picture of death by suicide even graver.

International comparability of data is also discussed. The information used in this paper, which reflects the official figures reported to WHO by member states, is based on death certificates signed by legally authorized personnel—usually doctors or police officers in the respective country. Usually these professionals have specific routines. How these routines differ between countries and regions, and how they influence suicide statistics, remains to be demonstrated through comparative studies of mortality statistics.

Moreover, it should be borne in mind that reporting of mortality statistics to WHO is subject to delays that vary from one country to the next. Accordingly, years for which data are available are not always the same. Data from 71% of the 90 countries (areas) included in the analysis covered the period 1995–2002. Around half (44 countries) had data for the year 2000 or later. Among these 44, most were in the European region. The remaining countries' data were from the period 1980–1994. After performing the analyses for the 90 countries (areas), we repeated the same analyses for the 63 countries (areas) in which the suicide data and mortality statistics were available for the year 1995. The results concerning suicide rates and the ranking of suicide as a cause of death were fairly similar in the two analyses (with a slightly higher global suicide rate for young people in the analysis for the year 1995).

During the period studied, different ICD classifications were used. This may have been an additional source of misclassification in the mortality statistics.

The mean suicide rate of 7.4/100,000 (10.5 for males and 4.1 for females) may be perceived as a reasonable estimate for the 15–19 age group and used as a basis for evaluating suicide rates among adolescents in different local communities.

In the calculation of suicide rates, the numbers of suicides in two large countries with more than 1,000 suicides in the 15–19 age group (Russia, with 2,883 cases in 2002; and USA, with 1,616 in 2000) accounted for 37.3% of the total, thus heavily influencing the mean rate. Interestingly, these two countries' suicide rates were markedly different. The Russian rate was 23.6/100,000, more than three times the mean (7.4), whereas that in the USA was 8.0, fairly close to the mean. Sri Lanka had an extraordinarily high suicide rate in the 15–19 age group: at 46.5/100,000, it was more than six times the mean rate. Unfortunately, data for recent years are not available for Sri Lanka.

Suicide rates for young people in the 15–19 age group are, as for other age groups, higher in males than in females. Young males' overall suicide rate was 2.6 times that of females. Exceptions were found in a number of non-European countries, like Sri Lanka, El Salvador, Cuba, Ecuador, and China, where suicide rates for females 15–19 years old exceeded those of males in the same age group. This fact urgently calls for further investigations.

Data from the latest 35-year period (1965–1999) show a marked difference in suicide rates between European and non-European countries. The high rates in non-European countries call for more attention. One reason for the lower suicide rates in European countries (although suicide rates in this region also vary widely from one country to another), beside cultural and psychosocial factors, may possibly be the physicians' awareness of the importance of adequately treating people with psychiatric disorders, psychosocial problems, and harmful stress.

However, this does not apply to the whole European region, since countries in transition show very high suicide rates, both for adults and for young people.

The fact that suicide rates are higher in males than in females has long been widely recognized. However, this study shows that suicide as a cause of death in the 15–19 age group is very similar in both sexes: 9.5% in males and 8.2% in females.

Suicide is one of the leading causes of death among young persons of both sexes. It is the leading cause of death in this age group after transport and other accidents and assault for males, and after transport and other accidents and neoplasms for females.

Scrutiny of the data for individual countries has revealed differences both in suicide rates and in the ranking of leading causes of death. These differences seem to be due to social, cultural and other factors, which call for further investigation.

In conclusion, suicide among young people is a major health problem in many societies, and preventive measures are strongly recommended (2).

References

1. Bertolote JM. Suicide in the world: an epidemiological overview, 1959–2000. In: Wasserman D, editor. *Suicide - an unnecessary death*. London: Dunitz; 2001. pp. 3–10.

2. Wasserman D. *Suicide - an unnecessary death*. London: Dunitz; 2001.

3. Mittendorfer Rutz E. Wasserman D. Trends in adolescent suicide mortality in the WHO European Region. *Eur Child Adolesc Psychiatry*. 2004;13:321–331.

4. La Vecchia C. Lucchini F. Levi F. Worldwide trends in suicide mortality, 1955–1989. *Acta Psychiatr Scand*. 1994;90:53–64.

5. Diekstra RFW. The epidemiology of suicide and parasuicide. *Arch Suicide Res*. 1996;2:1–29.

6. Schmidtke A. Weinracker B. Apter A. Suicide rates in the world: update. *Arch Suicide Res*. 1999;5:81–89.

7. Yang B. Lester D. Natural suicide rates in nations of the world. Short report. Crisis. 2004;25:187–188.

Chapter 4

Culture Plays A Role In Adolescent Suicide

In the United States, there is significant variability in suicidal ideation and behaviors among adolescents of different ethnic backgrounds. In adolescent populations, American Indian/Alaska Native youth tend to have highest rates of ideation and nonfatal suicidal behavior of all ethnic groups, followed by Latina/o and then African American and European American youth. Across ethnicities, nonfatal suicidal behavior is more common in girls than in boys, by an average ratio of 3 to 1. At the same time, the gender gap in rates of nonfatal suicidal behavior is most pronounced among youths of European American descent, and least pronounced among some American Indian youths (Canetto, 1997). For example, among Native Hawaiians and some American Indians (i.e., among Pueblo Indians but not Zuni Indians), adolescent males report similar rates of nonfatal suicidal behavior as adolescent females (Howard-Pitney, LaFromboise, Basil, September, & Johnson, 1992; Joe & Marcus, 2003; Yuen et al., 1996). American Indian youth have historically recorded the highest rates of suicide mortality, though there are significant variations in suicide mortality rates across tribes.

Across ethnicities, suicide is more common among boys than among girls, by an average ratio of 5 to 1 (Canetto & Lester, 1995). In recent decades, the gender gap in suicide mortality has been widening, especially in some U.S.

About This Chapter: Excerpted from "Advancing Prevention Research on the Role of Culture in Suicide Prevention," Sean Joe, MSW, PhD, Silvia Sara Canetto, PhD, and Daniel Romer, PhD, *Suicide & Life-Threatening Behavior*, June 2008, 38(3), 354–362. Copyright 2008 Guilford Publications, Inc. Reproduced with permission of Guilford Publications via Copyright Clearance Center.

❖ It's A Fact!!

Black Teens, Especially Girls, At High Risk For Suicide Attempts

Black American teens, especially females, may be at high risk for attempting suicide even if they have never been diagnosed with a mental disorder, according to researchers funded in part by the National Institute of Mental Health (NIMH). Their findings, based on responses from adolescent participants in the National Survey of American Life (NSAL), provide the first national estimates of suicidal thoughts and behaviors (ideation) and suicide attempts in 13 to 17-year-old black youth in the United States. The study was published in the March 2009 issue of the *Journal of the American Academy of Child and Adolescent Psychiatry*.

Background

Suicide is the third leading cause of death in all teens in the United States, according to the National Center for Health Statistics. Historically, black teens and young adults have lower suicide rates than white teens, but in recent decades, the suicide rate for black youth has increased dramatically.

The NSAL is a nationally representative, household survey of African Americans and blacks of Caribbean descent. From the NSAL households, 810 African American and 360 Caribbean black teens, ages 13–17, were randomly selected to complete the NSAL Adolescent survey (NSAL-A).

Findings From This Study

Sean Joe, Ph.D., LMSW, University of Michigan, and colleagues evaluated NSAL-A teens' responses to questions about suicidal ideation and nonfatal suicide attempts. According to the researchers, such attempts may occur up to 10–40 times more often than completed suicides and are important risk factors for future suicide.

According to the study, in a given year, African American teen girls are most likely to attempt suicide, followed by Caribbean teen girls, African American teen boys, and Caribbean teen boys.

However, Caribbean females in the study reported the highest rates for suicidal ideation, while Caribbean teen males reported the lowest rates for ideation and suicide attempts. This is in contrast to a previous NSAL report, which found that Caribbean adult males had the highest rates of suicide attempts among black Americans.

Also in contrast to previous studies, the researchers noted that youth from lower income households ($18,000–$31,999 annually) were least likely to report attempting suicide, while youth living in homes of modest means ($32,000–$54,999) were most likely.

Having a mental disorder was closely linked to attempted suicide among study participants. Teens with anxiety disorders were a highest risk. Despite this relationship, roughly half of teens who attempted suicide did not have or were never diagnosed with a mental disorder.

As in previous studies, teens living in the U.S. South and West appeared to be less at risk for attempted suicide than those living in the Northeast.

Overall, the researchers estimated that at some point before they reach 17 years of age, four percent of black teens, and more than seven percent of black teen females, will attempt suicide.

Reference

Joe S, Baser RS, Neighbors HW, Caldwell CH, S Jackson J. 12-Month and Lifetime Prevalence of Suicide Attempts Among Black Adolescents in the National Survey of American Life. *J Am Acad Child Adolesc Psychiatry*. 2009 Mar;48(3):271-82.

Source: Excerpted from "Black Teens, Especially Girls, at High Risk for Suicide Attempts, a Science Update from the National Institute of Mental Health, April 10, 2009.

ethnic minority groups (Centers for Disease Control and Prevention [CDC], 1998, 2004; Joe & Marcus, 2003; Substance Abuse and Mental Health Services Administration [SAMSHA], 2003). The widening gender gap is mostly due to increased suicide rates for ethnic minority boys since rates of suicide mortality among girls of all ethnic groups have remained stable. Historically, European American youths had higher rates of suicide than African American youths. In recent decades, however, suicide rates for African American male adolescents have increased more rapidly than suicide rates for European American male adolescents, such that the gap between the rates for these two groups is now narrower. The increase in African American male youth suicide has been particularly substantial in the South (CDC, 1998).

Longitudinal studies indicate that the variability in suicidal behaviors across ethnicities has become less pronounced in the last 20 years (Goldsmith, Pellmar, Kleinman, & Bunney, 2002; Mohler & Earls, 2001; Thompson, 2004); for example, rates of suicide among Hispanic and African American youths have become increasingly similar to those of European American youths (CDC, 1998, 2004; Joe & Marcus, 2003; SAMSHA, 2003). The "gender paradox" of suicidal behavior, however, persists (Canetto, 1997; Canetto & Lester, 1998), where males have higher suicide mortality and females have higher nonfatal suicidal behavior.

In addition to gender and ethnicity, other factors appear to be associated with risk for suicidal behavior among adolescents. One important such factor is sexual orientation. Young persons who identify as lesbian, gay, or bisexual are twice as likely as their heterosexual peers to have a history of suicidal behavior (Russell & Joyner, 2001). High rates of nonfatal suicidal behavior have been especially well documented among gay males (McDaniel, Purcell, & D'Augelli, 2001). Another factor is social class. Adolescents who engage in nonfatal suicidal behavior tend to be from lower socioeconomic strata, and low levels of parental education are associated with higher adolescent suicidal risk (Canetto, 1997).

Despite evidence of considerable ethnic variation in adolescent suicidal behavior, research has focused on youth of European American descent. This research has identified potential suicidal behavior risk factors for this population (Beautrais, 2003). Risk factors include a history of mental disorders, physical illness and functional impairment, and cultural permissibility; psychological and physical access to immediately lethal methods; and exposure to suicidal behavior (including a family history of suicidal behavior, recent suicidal behavior by a friend, and a person's own past suicidal episodes). Stressful life events, including turmoil and instability in important relationships, particularly in the parent-child relationship, appear to be precipitants of suicidal behavior in adolescents (Canetto, 1997; Evans, Hawton, & Rodham, 2004). However, the high or increasing rates of suicidal behavior of some ethnic minority adolescents, particularly ethnic minority boys, remain relatively unexplored.

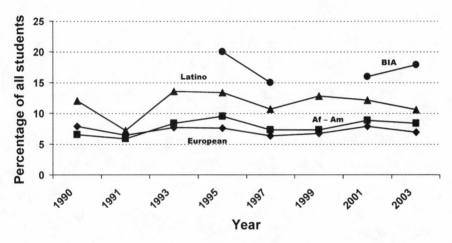

Figure 4.1. *Percentage of high school students who report suicidal behavior* by ethnicity, 1980–2003. (*At least one attempt during the 12 months preceding the survey. European and African American youth do not include Latinos). Source: Youth Risk Behavior Surveillance System (YRBSS) and Bureau of Indian Affairs (BIA) YRBSS.*

A key issue in adolescent suicidal behavior is that risk factors often impact boys and girls differently. On the one hand, similar risk factors are associated with different suicidal behaviors in boys and girls, specifically fatal suicidal behavior in boys and nonfatal suicidal behavior in girls. Relative to girls, boys seem protected from suicidal ideation and nonfatal suicidal behavior but more vulnerable to suicide mortality. On the other hand, different factors are sometimes associated with suicidal behavior in girls and boys. For example, mental disorders, depression, alcohol and substance abuse, and conduct disorders are most commonly associated with risk for suicidal ideation and behavior, both fatal and nonfatal, among European American adolescents. However, for European American girls, depression appears to be a better predictor of suicidal behavior than for boys, while alcohol and substance abuse and conduct disorders appear to be stronger correlates of suicidal behavior for European American boys than for girls. In recent years in the United States, sexual abuse is increasingly being recognized as a factor in girls' nonfatal suicidal behavior. Also, conflict with parents seems to create a unique vulnerability for girls' nonfatal suicidal behavior (Canetto, 1997).

References

Beautrais AL. Life course factors associated with suicidal behavior in young people. *American Behavioral Scientist*. 2003;46:1137–1156.

Canetto SS, Lester D. Gender and the primary prevention of suicide mortality. *Suicide and Life-Threatening Behavior*. 1995;25:58–69.

Canetto SS. Meanings of gender and suicidal behavior among adolescents. *Suicide and Life-Threatening Behavior*. 1997;27:339–351.

Centers for Disease Control and Prevention. Suicide among African-American youths—United States, 1980–1995. *Morbidity and Mortality Weekly Report*. 1998;47:193–196.

Centers for Disease Control and Prevention. *Youth risk behavior surveillance—United States*, 2003. Atlanta: Author; 2004.

Evans E, Hawton K, Rodham K. Factors associated with suicidal phenomena in adolescents: A systematic review of population-based studies. *Clinical Psychology Review*. 2004;24:957–979.

Goldsmith SK, Pellmar TC, Kleinman AM, Bunney WE. *Reducing suicide: A national imperative*. Washington, DC: Institute of Medicine, National Academies Press; 2002.

Howard-Pitney B, LaFromboise TD, Basil M, September B, Johnson M. Psychological and social indicators of suicide ideation and suicide attempts in Zuni adolescents. *Journal of Consulting and Clinical Psychology*. 1992;60:473–476.

Joe S, Marcus SC. Trends by race and gender in suicide attempts among U.S. adolescents, 1991–2001. *Psychiatric Services*. 2003;54:454.

McDaniel JS, Purcell D, D'Augelli AR. The relationship between sexual orientation and risk for suicide: Research findings and future directions for research and prevention. *Suicide and Life-Threatening Behavior.* 2001;31 Suppl:84–105.

Mohler B, Earls F. Trends in adolescent suicide: Misclassification bias? *American Journal of Public Health.* 2001;91:150–153.

Russell ST, Joyner K. Adolescent sexual orientation and suicide risk: Evidence from a national study. *American Journal of Public Health.* 2001;91:1276–1281.

Substance Abuse and Mental Health Services Administration. *Summary of findings from the 2000 National Household Survey on Drug Abuse* (DHHS Publication No. SMA 01- 3549, NHSDA Series: H-13). Rockville, MD: Author; 2003.

Thompson R. What can suicide researchers learn from African Americans? *American Journal of Public Health.* 2004;94:908.

Yuen N, Andrade N, Nahulu L, Makini G, McDermott JF, Danko G, et al. The rate and characteristics of suicide attempters in the Native Hawaiian adolescent population. *Suicide and Life-Threatening Behavior.* 1996;26:27–36.

Chapter 5

Facts About Suicide In Older Adults

Older Adults: Depression And Suicide Facts

How common is suicide among older adults?

Older Americans are disproportionately likely to die by suicide.

- Although they comprise only 12 percent of the U.S. population, people age 65 and older accounted for 16 percent of suicide deaths in 2004.

- 14.3 of every 100,000 people age 65 and older died by suicide in 2004, higher than the rate of about 11 per 100,000 in the general population.

- Non-Hispanic white men age 85 and older were most likely to die by suicide. They had a rate of 49.8 suicide deaths per 100,000 persons in that age group.

About This Chapter: This chapter begins with text excerpted from "Older Adults: Depression and Suicide Facts (Fact Sheet)," National Institute of Mental Health, 2007. The complete text of this document, including references, is available online at http://nimh .nih.gov/health/publications/older-adults-depression-and-suicide-facts-fact-sheet/index. shtml. Text under the heading "Prevention Of Depression And Suicide In Older Adults" is excerpted from "Community Integration for Older Adults with Mental Illnesses: Overcoming Barriers and Seizing Opportunities," National Mental Health Information Center, 2005. The complete text is available online at http://mentalhealth.samhsa.gov/ publications/allpubs/sma05-4018/sec3.asp.

✔ **Quick Tip**

IF YOU ARE IN CRISIS OR KNOW SOMEONE IN CRISIS AND NEED HELP RIGHT AWAY, call this toll-free number, available 24 hours a day, every day: 1-800-273-TALK (8255). You will reach the National Suicide Prevention Lifeline, a service available to anyone. You may call for yourself or for someone you care about. All calls are confidential.

Source: National Institute of Mental Health, 2007.

What role does depression play?

Depression, one of the conditions most commonly associated with suicide in older adults, is a widely under-recognized and undertreated medical illness. Studies show that many older adults who die by suicide—up to 75 percent—visited a physician within a month before death. These findings point to the urgency of improving detection and treatment of depression to reduce suicide risk among older adults.

- The risk of depression in the elderly increases with other illnesses and when ability to function becomes limited. Estimates of major depression in older people living in the community range from less than one percent to about five percent, but rises to 13.5 percent in those who require home healthcare and to 11.5 percent in elderly hospital patients.

- An estimated five million have subsyndromal depression, symptoms that fall short of meeting the full diagnostic criteria for a disorder. Subsyndromal depression is especially common among older persons and is associated with an increased risk of developing major depression.

Isn't depression just part of aging?

Depressive disorder is not a normal part of aging. Emotional experiences of sadness, grief, response to loss, and temporary "blue" moods are normal. Persistent depression that interferes significantly with ability to function is not.

Health professionals may mistakenly think that persistent depression is an acceptable response to other serious illnesses and the social and financial hardships that often accompany aging—an attitude often shared by older people themselves. This contributes to low rates of diagnosis and treatment in older adults.

Depression can and should be treated when it occurs at the same time as other medical illnesses. Untreated depression can delay recovery or worsen the outcome of these other illnesses.

What are the treatments for depression in older adults?

Antidepressant medications or psychotherapy, or a combination of the two, can be effective treatments for late-life depression.

Antidepressant medications affect brain chemicals called neurotransmitters. For example, medications called SSRIs (selective serotonin reuptake inhibitors) affect the neurotransmitter serotonin. Different medications may affect different neurotransmitters.

Some older adults may find that newer antidepressant medications, including SSRIs, have fewer side effects than older medications, which include tricyclic antidepressants and monoamine oxidase inhibitors (MAOIs). However, others may find that these older medications work well for them.

It's important to be aware that there are several medications for depression, that different medications work for different people, and that it takes four to eight weeks for the medications to work. If one medication doesn't help, research shows that a different antidepressant might.

Also, older adults experiencing depression for the first time should talk to their doctors about continuing medication even if their symptoms have disappeared with treatment. Studies showed that patients age 70 and older who became symptom-free and continued to take their medication for two more years were 60 percent less likely to relapse than those who discontinued their medications.

In psychotherapy, people interact with a specially trained health professional to deal with depression, thoughts of suicide, and other problems. Research shows that certain types of psychotherapy are effective treatments for late-life depression.

For many older adults, especially those who are in good physical health, combining psychotherapy with antidepressant medication appears to provide the most benefit. A study showed that about 80 percent of older adults with depression recovered with this kind of combined treatment and had lower recurrence rates than with psychotherapy or medication alone.

Another study of depressed older adults with physical illnesses and problems with memory and thinking showed that combined treatment was no more effective than medication alone. Research can help further determine which older adults appear to be most likely to benefit from a combination of medication and psychotherapy or from either treatment alone.

❖ It's A Fact!!
Suicide In The Elderly

Older adults do not usually seek treatment for mental health problems. Family and friends can play an important role in prevention. Some warning signs include the following:

- Loss of interest in things or activities that are usually found enjoyable
- Cutting back social interaction, self-care, and grooming
- Breaking medical regimens (such as going off diets, prescriptions)
- Experiencing or expecting a significant personal loss (spouse or other)
- Feeling hopeless and/or worthless
- Putting affairs in order, giving things away, or making changes in wills
- Stock-piling medication or obtaining other lethal means

Other clues are a preoccupation with death or a lack of concern about personal safety. Remarks such as "This is the last time that you'll see me" or "I won't be needing anymore appointments" should raise concern. The most significant indicator is an expression of suicidal intent.

Despite the availability of safe and effective treatments, late-life mood disorders remain a large problem. One reason for this may be that the public sees depression and suicide as normal aspects of aging. A sizable portion of the population views youth suicide as a greater tragedy than late-life suicide. This way of thinking works against effective outreach to the elderly and efforts to understand and treat their conditions. The health care system is not meeting the needs of many elderly, and discriminatory coverage and reimbursement policies for mental health care are significant barriers to treatment.

Are some ethnic/racial groups at higher risk of suicide?

For every 100,000 people age 65 and older in each of the ethnic/racial groups below, the following number died by suicide in 2004:

- Non-Hispanic Whites: 15.8 per 100,000
- Asian and Pacific Islanders: 10.6 per 100,000
- Hispanics: 7.9 per 100,000
- Non-Hispanic Blacks: 5.0 per 100,000

Most service agencies aim for self-sufficiency in terms of individual capability and safety. This commitment to independence may cause community agencies to let the client or patient control information, such as alerting relatives or involving other available services. In this way, the elder with thoughts of suicide can filter and control the flow of information about his or her condition.

Taking action to help can include getting the word out (that someone is in danger of committing suicide) into the stream of communication, letting others know about it, breaking what could be called a fatal secret, talking to the person, talking to others, offering help, getting loved ones interested and responsive, creating action around the person, showing response, indicating interest, and, if possible, showing deep concern.

Options for prevention can contain various strategies, including limiting access to firearms and reducing the inappropriate use of sedative medications. Most importantly, educational programs for primary health care providers on the identification and treatment of late-life depression can be a vital component of lowering suicide rates. Evidence shows that most elderly suicide victims visit their physician shortly before dying. In fact, over 70% of older patients who die by suicide visit their primary care physician within a month of their death. Most of these clients are not diagnosed with a psychiatric disorder and do not seek mental health services.

Source: Excerpted from "AAMFT Consumer Update: Suicide in the Elderly," Copyright 2002 American Association for Marriage and Family Therapy. Reproduced with permission of the American Association for Marriage and Family Therapy, via Copyright Clearance Center.

Prevention Of Depression And Suicide In Older Adults

Depression in older adults is a serious public health concern. Furthermore, more than two-fifths of older adults with schizophrenia show signs of clinical depression. A recent study in the *American Journal of Geriatric Psychiatry* revealed that depressive states that fall below the clinical threshold are frequent and persistent in older adults and are associated with distress and disability. Investigators also found that individuals who initially had less severe forms of depression were more likely to develop major depression than individuals who had not been depressed.

Risk factors for late-life depression in older adults include female gender, widowhood, physical illness or impaired function, heavy use of alcohol, and absence of a support network. Depression in older adults is associated with increased health care use, poor quality of life, and risk for suicide.

Both support groups and peer counseling have been shown to be effective for older adults at risk for depression. Bereavement support groups, in particular, can help improve mental health status for widows and widowers. Evaluation of a program run by the American Association of Retired People (AARP) called the Widowed Persons Service, which pairs new widows with a widow who can provide emotional support and practical assistance, found that women receiving the intervention recovered more quickly and experienced fewer depressive symptoms than those who did not participate.

Peer counselor prevention focuses on early detection, or self-detection, and referral to care before the illness becomes acute. The Skagit Community Mental Health Center in Washington State has published a training manual for older adult peer counselors. The use of older adult consumer counselors provides a unique opportunity for older consumers to share with their peers, who will talk to them from firsthand experience about the symptoms of mental illnesses and substance abuse disorders and the fact that treatment works.

Chapter 6

Firearms And Suicide

This past June [2008], in a five-to-four decision in District of Columbia v. Heller, the Supreme Court struck down a ban on handgun ownership in the nation's capital and ruled that the District's law requiring all firearms in the home to be locked violated the Second Amendment. But the Supreme Court's finding of a Second Amendment right to have a handgun in the home does not mean that it is a wise decision to own a gun or to keep it easily accessible. Deciding whether to own a gun entails balancing potential benefits and risks. One of the risks for which the empirical evidence is strongest, and the risk whose death toll is greatest, is that of completed suicide.

In 2005, the most recent year for which mortality data are available, suicide was the second-leading cause of death among Americans 40 years of age or younger. Among Americans of all ages, more than half of all suicides are gun suicides. In 2005, an average of 46 Americans per day committed suicide with a firearm, accounting for 53% of all completed suicides. Gun suicide during this period accounted for 40% more deaths than gun homicide.

About This Chapter: Text in this chapter is from "Guns and Suicide in the United States," by Matthew Miller, MD, ScD, and David Hemenway, PhD. *New England Journal of Medicine*, 359;10, 989–991, September 4, 2008. Copyright © 2008 Massachusetts Medical Society. All rights reserved. Reprinted with permission. Dr. Miller is the associate director and Dr. Hemenway the director of the Harvard Injury Control Research Center, Harvard School of Public Health, Boston. No potential conflict of interest relevant to this article was reported.

Why might the availability of firearms increase the risk of suicide in the United States? First, many suicidal acts—one third to four fifths of all suicide attempts, according to studies—are impulsive. Among people who made near-lethal suicide attempts, for example, 24% took less than five minutes between the decision to kill themselves and the actual attempt, and 70% took less than one hour.

Second, many suicidal crises are self-limiting. Such crises are often caused by an immediate stressor, such as the breakup of a romantic relationship, the loss of a job, or a run-in with police. As the acute phase of the crisis passes, so does the urge to attempt suicide.

Third, guns are common in the United States (more than one third of U.S. households contain a firearm) and are lethal. A suicide attempt with a firearm rarely affords a second chance. Attempts involving drugs or cutting, which account for more than 90% of all suicidal acts, prove fatal far less often.

The empirical evidence linking suicide risk in the United States to the presence of firearms in the home is compelling. There are at least a dozen U.S. case–control studies in the peer-reviewed literature, all of which have found that a gun in the home is associated with an increased risk of suicide. The increase in risk is large, typically two to 10 times that in homes without guns, depending on the sample population (for example, adolescents vs. older adults) and on the way in which the firearms were stored. The association between guns in the home and the risk of suicide is due entirely to a large increase in the risk of suicide by firearm that is not counterbalanced by a reduced risk of nonfirearm suicide. Moreover, the increased risk of suicide is not explained by increased psychopathologic characteristics, suicidal ideation, or suicide attempts among members of gun-owning households.

☞ **Remember!!**
The temporary nature and fleeting sway of many suicidal crises is evident in the fact that more than 90% of people who survive a suicide attempt, including attempts that were expected to be lethal (such as shooting oneself in the head or jumping in front of a train), do not go on to die by suicide. Indeed, recognizing the self-limiting nature of suicidal crises, penal and psychiatric institutions restrict access to lethal means for persons identified as potentially suicidal.

Three additional findings from the case-control studies are worth noting. The higher risk of suicide in homes with firearms applies not only to the gun owner but also to the gun owner's spouse and children. The presence of a gun in the home, no matter how the gun is stored, is a risk factor for completed suicide. And there is a hierarchy of suicide risk consistent with a dose-response relationship. How household guns are stored matters especially for young people—for example, one study found that adolescent suicide was four times as likely in homes with a loaded, unlocked firearm as in homes where guns were stored unloaded and locked.

Many ecologic studies covering multiple regions, states, or cities in the United States have also shown a strong association between rates of household gun ownership and rates of completed suicide—attributable, as found in the case–control studies, to the strong association between gun prevalence and gun suicide, without a counterbalancing association between gun-ownership levels and rates of nongun suicide. We [the authors of this study] recently examined the relationship between rates of household gun ownership and suicide in each of the 50 states for the period between 2000 and 2002. We used data on gun ownership from a large telephone survey (of more than 200,000 respondents) and controlled for rates of poverty, urbanization, unemployment, mental illness, and drug and alcohol dependence and abuse. Among men, among women, and in every age group (including children), states with higher rates of household gun ownership had higher rates of firearm suicide and overall suicides. There was no association between firearm-ownership rates and nonfirearm suicides. To illustrate the main findings, we presented data for the 15 states with the highest levels of household gun ownership matched with the six states with the lowest levels (using only six so that the populations in both groups of states would be approximately equal). In the table, the findings are updated for 2001 through 2005.

The recent Supreme Court decision may lead to higher rates of gun owner-ship. Such an outcome would increase the incidence of suicide. Two comple-mentary approaches are available to physicians to help counter this possibility: to try to reduce the number of suicide attempts (for example, by recognizing and treating mental illness) and to try to reduce the probability that suicide attempts will prove fatal (for example, by reducing access to lethal means).

Many U.S. physicians, from primary care practitioners to psychiatrists, focus exclusively on the first approach. Yet international experts have concluded that restriction of access to lethal means is one of the few suicide-prevention policies with proven effectiveness.

In our experience, many clinicians who care deeply about preventing suicide are unfamiliar with the evidence linking guns to suicide. Too many seem to believe that anyone who is serious enough about suicide to use a gun would find an equally effective means if a gun were not available. This belief is invalid.

Table 6.1. Data On Suicides In States With The Highest And Lowest Rates Of Gun Ownership, 2001–2005.*

Variable	States with the Highest Rate of Gun Ownership	States with the Lowest Rate of Gun Ownership	Ratio of Mortality Rates
Person-years	195 million	200 million	
Percent of households with guns	47	15	
Male			
No. of firearm suicides	14,365	3,971	3.7
No. of nonfirearm suicides	6,573	6,781	1.0
Total no.	20,938	10,752	2.0
Female			
No. of firearm suicides	2,212	286	7.9
No. of nonfirearm suicides	2,599	2,478	1.1
Total no.	4,811	2,764	1.8

*The states with the highest rates of gun ownership included here are Wyoming, South Dakota, Alaska, West Virginia, Montana, Arkansas, Mississippi, Idaho, North Dakota, Alabama, Kentucky, Wisconsin, Louisiana, Tennessee, and Utah. The states with the lowest rates of gun ownership included here are Hawaii, Massachusetts, Rhode Island, New Jersey, Connecticut, and New York. Data on gun ownership are from the 2001 Behavioral Risk Factor Surveillance System. Data on suicides are from the Centers for Disease Control and Prevention Web-Based Injury Statistics Query and Reporting System.

Physicians and other health care providers who care for suicidal patients should be able to assess whether people at risk for suicide have access to a firearm or other lethal means and to work with patients and their families to limit access to those means until suicidal feelings have passed. A website of the Harvard Injury Control Research Center can help physicians and others in this effort (www.hsph.harvard.edu/means-matter). Effective suicide prevention should focus not only on a patient's psychological condition but also on the availability of lethal means—which can make the difference between life and death.

References

Hemenway D. *Private guns, public health*. Ann Arbor: University of Michigan Press, 2004.

Simon OR, Swann AC, Powell KE, Potter LB, Kresnow MJ, O'Carroll PW. Characteristics of impulsive suicide attempts and attempters. *Suicide Life Threat Behav* 2001;32:Suppl:49-59.

Miller M, Hemenway D. The relationship between firearms and suicide: a review of the literature. *Aggress Violent Behav* 1999;4:59-75.

Miller M, Lippmann SJ, Azrael D, Hemenway D. Household firearm ownership and rates of suicide across the 50 United States. *J Trauma* 2007;62:1029-1035.

Mann JJ, Apter A, Bertolote J, et al. Suicide prevention strategies: a systematic review. *JAMA* 2005;294:2064-2074.

Chapter 7

Attitudes About Mental Health

Nationally representative surveys have tracked public attitudes about mental illness since the 1950s. To permit comparisons over time, several surveys of the 1970s and the 1990s phrased questions exactly as they had been asked in the 1950s.

In the 1950s, the public viewed mental illness as a stigmatized condition and displayed an unscientific understanding of mental illness. Survey respondents typically were not able to identify individuals as "mentally ill" when presented with vignettes of individuals who would have been said to be mentally ill according to the professional standards of the day. The public was not particularly skilled at distinguishing mental illness from ordinary unhappiness and worry and tended to see only extreme forms of behavior—namely psychosis—as mental illness. Mental illness carried great social stigma, especially linked with fear of unpredictable and violent behavior.

By 1996, a modern survey revealed that Americans had achieved greater scientific understanding of mental illness. But the increases in knowledge did not defuse social stigma. The public learned to define mental illness and

About This Chapter: This chapter includes text excerpted from "Chapter 1: Introduction and Themes," *Mental Health: A Report of the Surgeon General*, Office of the Surgeon General, U.S. Department of Health and Human Services, 1999; accessed in November 2009. Despite the older date of this document, the background information about potential sources of stigma related to mental illness is still pertinent. The complete text of this document, including references, is available at http://www.surgeongeneral.gov/library/mentalhealth/chapter1/sec1.html.

to distinguish it from ordinary worry and unhappiness. It expanded its definition of mental illness to encompass anxiety, depression, and other mental disorders. The public attributed mental illness to a mix of biological abnormalities and vulnerabilities to social and psychological stress. Yet, in comparison with the 1950s, the public's perception of mental illness more frequently incorporated violent behavior. This was primarily true among those who defined mental illness to include psychosis (a view held by about one-third of the entire sample). Thirty-one percent of this group mentioned violence in its descriptions of mental illness, in comparison with 13 percent in the 1950s. In other words, the perception of people with psychosis as being dangerous is stronger today than in the past.

✤ It's A Fact!!

Stigmatization of people with mental disorders has persisted throughout history. It is manifested by bias, distrust, stereotyping, fear, embarrassment, anger, and/or avoidance. Stigma leads others to avoid living, socializing or working with, renting to, or employing people with mental disorders, especially severe disorders such as schizophrenia. It reduces patients' access to resources and opportunities (for example, housing, jobs) and leads to low self-esteem, isolation, and hopelessness. It deters the public from seeking, and wanting to pay for, care. In its most overt and egregious form, stigma results in outright discrimination and abuse. More tragically, it deprives people of their dignity and interferes with their full participation in society.

The 1996 survey also probed how perceptions of those with mental illness varied by diagnosis. The public was more likely to consider an individual with schizophrenia as having mental illness than an individual with depression. All of them were distinguished reasonably well from a worried and unhappy individual who did not meet professional criteria for a mental disorder. The desire for social distance was consistent with this hierarchy.

Why is stigma so strong despite better public understanding of mental illness? The answer appears to be fear of violence: people with mental illness, especially those with psychosis, are perceived to be more violent than in the past.

This finding begs yet another question: are people with mental disorders truly more violent? Research supports some public concerns, but the overall likelihood of violence is low. The greatest risk of violence is from those who have dual diagnoses, that is, individuals who have a mental disorder as well as a substance abuse disorder. There is a small elevation in risk of violence from individuals with severe mental disorders (for example, psychosis), especially if they are noncompliant with their medication. Yet the risk of violence is much less for a stranger than for a family member or person who is known to the person with mental illness. In fact, there is very little risk of violence or harm to a stranger from casual contact with an individual who has a mental disorder. Because the average person is ill-equipped to judge whether someone who is behaving erratically has any of these disorders, alone or in combination, the natural tendency is to be wary. Yet, to put this all in perspective, the overall contribution of mental disorders to the total level of violence in society is exceptionally small.

Because most people should have little reason to fear violence from those with mental illness, even in its most severe forms, why is fear of violence so entrenched? Most speculations focus on media coverage and deinstitutionalization. One series of surveys found that selective media reporting reinforced the public's stereotypes linking violence and mental illness and encouraged people to distance themselves from those with mental disorders. And yet, deinstitutionalization made this distancing impossible over the 40 years as the population of state and county mental hospitals was reduced from a high of about 560,000 in 1955 to well below 100,000 by the 1990s.

✤ It's A Fact!!

In colonial times in the United States, people with mental illness were described as "lunatics" and were largely cared for by families. There was no concerted effort to treat mental illness until urbanization in the early 19th century created a societal problem that previously had been relegated to families scattered among small rural communities. Social policy assumed the form of isolated asylums where persons with mental illness were administered the reigning treatments of the era. Throughout the history of institutionalization in asylums (later renamed mental hospitals), reformers strove to improve treatment and curtail abuse. Several waves of reform culminated in the deinstitutionalization movement that began in the 1950s with the goal of shifting patients and care to the community.

Some advocates of deinstitutionalization expected stigma to be reduced with community care and commonplace exposure. Stigma might have been greater today had not public education resulted in a more scientific understanding of mental illness.

Stigma And Seeking Help For Mental Disorders

Nearly two-thirds of all people with diagnosable mental disorders do not seek treatment. Stigma surrounding the receipt of mental health treatment is among the many barriers that discourage people from seeking treatment. Concern about stigma appears to be heightened in rural areas in relation to larger towns or cities. Stigma also disproportionately affects certain age groups, as explained in the chapters on children and older people.

The surveys cited above concerning evolving public attitudes about mental illness also monitored how people would cope with, and seek treatment for, mental illness if they became symptomatic. (The term "nervous breakdown" was used in lieu of the term "mental illness" in the 1996 survey to allow for comparisons with the surveys in the 1950s and 1970s.) The 1996 survey found that people were likelier than in the past to approach mental illness by coping with, rather than by avoiding, the problem. They also were more likely now to want informal social supports (for example, self-help groups). Those who now sought formal support increasingly preferred counselors, psychologists, and social workers.

Stigma And Paying For Mental Disorder Treatment

Another manifestation of stigma is reflected in the public's reluctance to pay for mental health services. Public willingness to pay for mental health treatment, particularly through insurance premiums or taxes, has been assessed largely through public opinion polls. Members of the public report a greater willingness to pay for insurance coverage for individuals with severe mental disorders, such as schizophrenia and depression, rather than for less severe conditions such as worry and unhappiness. While the public generally appears to support paying for treatment, its support diminishes upon the realization that higher taxes or premiums would be necessary. In the lexicon of survey research, the willingness to pay for mental illness treatment services is considered to be "soft." The public generally ranks insurance coverage for mental disorders below that for somatic disorders.

Reducing Stigma

There is likely no simple or single panacea to eliminate the stigma associated with mental illness. Stigma was expected to abate with increased knowledge of mental illness, but just the opposite occurred: stigma in some ways intensified over the past 40 years even though understanding improved. Knowledge of mental illness appears by itself insufficient to dispel stigma. Broader knowledge may be warranted, especially to redress public fears. Research is beginning to demonstrate that negative perceptions about severe mental illness can be lowered by furnishing empirically based information on the association between

❖ It's A Fact!!

One reason the public continues to emphasize the difference between mental and physical health is embedded in language. Common parlance continues to use the term "physical" to distinguish some forms of health and illness from "mental" health and illness. People continue to see mental and physical as separate functions when, in fact, mental functions (for example, memory) are physical as well. Likewise, mental disorders are reflected in physical changes in the brain. Physical changes in the brain often trigger physical changes in other parts of the body too. The racing heart, dry mouth, and sweaty palms that accompany a terrifying nightmare are all orchestrated by the brain.

Instead of dividing physical from mental health, the more appropriate and neutral distinction is between "mental" and "somatic" health. Somatic is a medical term that derives from the Greek word soma for the body. Mental health refers to the successful performance of mental functions in terms of thought, mood, and behavior. Mental disorders are those health conditions in which alterations in mental functions are paramount. Somatic conditions are those in which alterations in nonmental functions predominate.

While the brain carries out all mental functions, it also carries out some somatic functions, such as movement, touch, and balance. That is why not all brain diseases are mental disorders. For example, a stroke causes a lesion in the brain that may produce disturbances of movement, such as paralysis of limbs. When such symptoms predominate in a patient, the stroke is considered a somatic condition. But when a stroke mainly produces alterations of thought, mood, or behavior, it is considered a mental condition (for example, dementia). The point is that a brain disease can be seen as a mental disorder or a somatic disorder depending on the functions it perturbs.

violence and severe mental illness. Overall approaches to stigma reduction involve programs of advocacy, public education, and contact with persons with mental illness through schools and other societal institutions.

Another way to eliminate stigma is to find causes and effective treatments for mental disorders. History suggests this to be true. Neurosyphilis and pellagra are illustrative of mental disorders for which stigma has receded. In the early part of the 20th century, about 20 percent of those admitted to mental hospitals had "general paresis," later identified as tertiary syphilis. This advanced stage of syphilis occurs when the bacterium invades the brain and causes neurological deterioration (including psychosis), paralysis, and death. The discoveries of an infectious etiology and of penicillin led to the virtual elimination of neurosyphilis. Similarly, when pellagra was traced to a nutrient deficiency, and nutritional supplementation with niacin was introduced, the condition was eventually eradicated in the developed world. Pellagra's victims with delirium had been placed in mental hospitals early in the 20th century before its etiology was clarified. Although no one has documented directly the reduction of public stigma toward these conditions over the early and later parts of the century, disease eradication through widespread acceptance of treatment (and its cost) offers indirect proof.

Ironically, these examples also illustrate a more unsettling consequence: that the mental health field was adversely affected when causes and treatments were identified. As advances were achieved, each condition was transferred from the mental health field to another medical specialty. For instance, dominion over syphilis was moved to dermatology, internal medicine, and neurology upon advances in etiology and treatment. Dominion over hormone-related mental disorders was moved to endocrinology under similar circumstances. The consequence of this transformation, according to historian Gerald Grob, is that the mental health field became over the years the repository for mental disorders whose etiology was unknown. This left the mental health field "vulnerable to accusations by their medical brethren that psychiatry was not part of medicine, and that psychiatric practice rested on superstition and myth."

These historical examples signify that stigma dissipates for individual disorders once advances render them less disabling, infectious, or disfiguring. Yet the stigma surrounding other mental disorders not only persists but may be inadvertently reinforced by leaving to mental health care only those behavioral conditions without known causes or cures. To point this out is not intended to imply that advances in mental health should be halted; rather, advances should be nurtured and heralded. The purpose here is to explain some of the historical origins of the chasm between the health and mental health fields.

As stigma abates, a transformation in public attitudes should occur. People should become eager to seek care. They should become more willing to absorb its cost. And, most importantly, they should become far more receptive to the messages that mental health and mental illness are part of the mainstream of health, and they are a concern for all people.

☞ Remember!!

Stigma must be overcome. Research that will continue to yield increasingly effective treatments for mental disorders promises to be an effective antidote. When people understand that mental disorders are not the result of moral failings or limited will power, but are legitimate illnesses that are responsive to specific treatments, much of the negative stereotyping may dissipate. Still, fresh approaches to disseminate research information and, thus, to counter stigma need to be developed and evaluated. Social science research has much to contribute to the development and evaluation of anti-stigma programs.

Part Two

Mental Health Disorders
And Life-Threatening Behaviors
Linked To Suicide Risk

Chapter 8

Depression: A Key Risk For Suicide

Depression Is Common

Lately Lindsay hasn't felt like herself. Her friends have noticed it, too. Kia was surprised when Lindsay turned down her invitation to go to the mall last Saturday. There was really no reason not to go, but Lindsay just didn't feel like it. Instead, she spent most of Saturday sleeping.

Staying in more than usual isn't the only change in Lindsay. She's always been a really good student. But over the past couple of months her grades have fallen and she has trouble concentrating. She forgot to turn in a paper that was due and is having a hard time getting motivated to study for her finals.

Lindsay feels tired all the time but has difficulty falling asleep. She's gained weight too. When her mother asks her what's wrong, Lindsay just feels like crying. But she doesn't know why. Nothing particularly bad has happened. Yet Lindsay feels sad all the time and can't shake it.

Lindsay may not realize it yet, but she is depressed.

Depression is very common and affects as many as one in eight people in their teen years. Depression affects people of every color, race, economic status, or age; however, it does seem to affect more girls than guys.

About This Chapter: "Depression," October 2007, reprinted with permission from www .kidshealth.org. Copyright © 2007 The Nemours Foundation. This information was provided by KidsHealth, one of the largest resources online for medically reviewed health information written for parents, kids, and teens. For more articles like this one, visit www .KidsHealth.org, or www.TeensHealth.org.

How Do People Respond To Someone Who's Depressed?

Sometimes friends or family members recognize that someone is depressed. They may respond with love, kindness, or support, hoping that the sadness will soon pass. They may offer to listen if the person wants to talk. If the depressed feeling doesn't pass with a little time, friends or loved ones may encourage the person to get help from a doctor, therapist, or counselor.

But not everyone recognizes depression when it happens to someone they know. Some people don't really understand about depression. For example, they may react to a depressed person's low energy with criticism, yelling at the person for acting lazy or not trying harder. Some people mistakenly believe that depression is just an attitude or a mood that a person can shake off. It's not that easy.

❧ It's A Fact!!

Self-Reflection May Lead Independently To Creativity And Depression

With major depressive disorder eight to 10 times more prevalent in writers and artists than in the general population, mental health researchers and practitioners have long linked creativity with a higher risk for depression.

However, a study in the June [2005] issue of *Emotion* (Vol. 5, No. 2) suggests that self-reflective rumination—a focus on the self and one's feelings—may explain artists' tendency toward depression, taking the blame off creativity itself.

"Depression is associated with inactivity, difficulty concentrating and lying in bed, which seems contrary to creativity," says study co-author Jutta Joormann, PhD, a Stanford University researcher. "But depressed people are more likely to ruminate, making depression act as an intermediary variable," given that rumination can also lead individuals to generate a large number of ideas and, in turn, artistic endeavors.

To reach this finding, Syracuse University psychology professor Paul Verhaeghen, PhD, Joormann and their colleagues instructed 99 undergraduates to complete questionnaires measuring current and past depressive symptoms, creative interests and self-reflective rumination. The students—who were culled from introductory psychology classes, fine arts classes, an arts and sciences honors

Sometimes even people who are depressed don't take their condition seriously enough. Some people feel that they are weak in some way because they are depressed. This is wrong—and it can even be harmful if it causes people to hide their depression and avoid getting help.

Occasionally, when depression causes physical symptoms (things like headaches or other stress-related problems), a person may see a doctor. Once in a while, even a well-meaning doctor may not realize a person is depressed, and just treat the physical symptoms.

Why Do People Get Depressed?

There is no single cause for depression. Many factors play a role including genetics, environment, life events, medical conditions, and the way people react to things that happen in their lives.

---

program, and a campus writers group—also participated in two creative behavior tests that measure fluency of imagination and originality.

The researchers found no direct link between depression and creativity. However, self-reflection was correlated with both an increased risk for depression and an interest in, and talent for, creative behavior.

Joormann suggests that people most likely to have the blues are also those most likely to express them.

However, Joormann notes that the study does not explain all of the variance of creative behavior since she and her colleagues used only a sample of college students.

In future studies, Verhaeghen and his colleagues aim to expand their subject pool beyond college students to established artists and nonartists. They may also induce subjects to self-ruminate. Future findings could even inform treatment for depression, possibly indicating clinicians could use imagination, role-playing and other such techniques to reduce people's self-reflective tendencies, Joormann says.

"Knowing that people with depression are more prone to self-rumination and creativity may be a good resource to use in therapy," she says.

Genetics: Research shows that depression runs in families and that some people inherit genes that make it more likely for them to get depressed. Not everyone who has the genetic makeup for depression gets depressed, though. And many people who have no family history of depression have the condition. So although genes are one factor, they aren't the single cause of depression.

Life Events: The death of a family member, friend, or pet can go beyond normal grief and sometimes lead to depression. Other difficult life events, such as when parents divorce, separate, or remarry, can trigger depression. Even events like moving or changing schools can be emotionally challenging enough that a person becomes depressed.

✤ **It's A Fact!!**

Suicidal Thinking May Be Predicted Among Certain Teens With Depression

Certain circumstances may predict suicidal thinking or behavior among teens with treatment-resistant major depression who are undergoing second-step treatment, according to an analysis of data from a study funded by the National Institute of Mental Health (NIMH). The study was published online ahead of print February 17, 2009, in the *American Journal of Psychiatry*.

In the Treatment of SSRI-resistant Depression in Adolescents (TORDIA) study, 334 teens who did not get well after taking a type of antidepressant called a selective serotonin reuptake inhibitor (SSRI) before the trial were randomly assigned to one of four treatments for 12 weeks:

- Switch to another SSRI

- Switch to venlafaxine (Effexor), a different type of antidepressant

- Switch to another SSRI and add cognitive behavioral therapy (CBT), a type of psychotherapy

- Switch to venlafaxine and add CBT

Results of the trial were previously reported in February 2008. They showed that teens who received combination therapy, with either type of antidepressant, were more likely to get well than those on medication alone.

Family And Social Environment: For some teens, a negative, stressful, or unhappy family atmosphere can affect their self-esteem and lead to depression. This can also include high-stress living situations such as poverty, homelessness, and violence in the family, relationships, or community.

Substance use and abuse also can cause chemical changes in the brain that affect mood—alcohol and some drugs are known to have depressant effects. The negative social and personal consequences of substance abuse also can lead to severe unhappiness and depression.

Medical Conditions: Certain medical conditions can affect hormone balance and therefore have an effect on mood. Some conditions, such as hypothyroidism,

Using data from spontaneous reports by the participants and from systematic assessment by clinicians, David Brent, MD, of the Western Psychiatric Institute and Clinic, and colleagues aimed to identify characteristics or circumstances that may predict whether a teen is likely to have suicidal thoughts or behavior during treatment. Nearly 60 percent of TORDIA participants had suicidal thinking or behavior at the beginning of the trial.

Fifty-eight suicidal events—which include serious suicidal thinking or a recent suicide attempt—occurred in 48 participants during the trial, most of which happened early in the trial. The researchers found that teens who had higher levels of suicidal thinking, higher levels of parent-child conflict, and who used drugs or alcohol at the trial's beginning were more likely to experience a suicidal event during treatment and less likely to respond to treatment. They were also less likely to have completed treatment.

"These new data may contribute to developing more targeted and individualized interventions." said NIMH co-author Benedetto Vitiello, MD. "If we can know which teens may be more susceptible to suicidal thinking and behavior, we are better able to tailor safer treatments for them."

"Because the suicidal events tended to happen early in the treatment process, interventions that address safety, emotion regulation and family conflict should be some of the first to be implemented," concluded Dr. Brent. "With this data, we are in a better position to design future interventions that could lessen the risks of suicide even further among this vulnerable population."

Source: Excerpted from "Suicidal Thinking May Be Predicted Among Certain Teens with Depression," a Science Update from the National Institute of Mental Health, February 17, 2009.

are known to cause a depressed mood in some people. When these medical conditions are diagnosed and treated by a doctor, the depression usually disappears.

For some teens, undiagnosed learning disabilities might block school success, hormonal changes might affect mood, or physical illness might present challenges or setbacks.

What Happens In The Brain When Someone Is Depressed?

Depression involves the brain's delicate chemistry—specifically, it involves chemicals called neurotransmitters. These chemicals help send messages between nerve cells in the brain. Certain neurotransmitters regulate mood, and if they run low, people can become depressed, anxious, and stressed. Stress also can affect the balance of neurotransmitters and lead to depression.

Sometimes, a person may experience depression without being able to point to any particular sad or stressful event. People who have a genetic predisposition to depression may be more prone to the imbalance of neurotransmitter activity that is part of depression.

Medications that doctors use to treat depression work by helping to restore the proper balance of neurotransmitters.

Types Of Depression

For some people, depression can be intense and occur in bouts that last for weeks at a time. For others, depression can be less severe but can linger at a low level for years.

Doctors who treat depression distinguish between these two types of depression. They call the more severe, short-lasting type major depression, and the longer-lasting but less severe form dysthymia (pronounced: diss-thy-me-uh).

A third form of depression that doctors may diagnose is called adjustment disorder with depressed mood. This diagnosis refers to a depressive reaction to a specific life event (such as a death, divorce, or other loss), when adjusting to the loss takes longer than the normally expected timeframe or is more severe than expected and interferes with the person's daily activities.

Bipolar disorder (also sometimes called manic depressive illness) is another depressive condition that involves periods of major depression mixed with periods of mania. Mania is the term for abnormally high mood and extreme bursts of unusual activity or energy.

What Are The Symptoms Of Depression?

Symptoms that people have when they're depressed can include:

- depressed mood or sadness most of the time (for what may seem like no reason);
- lack of energy and feeling tired all the time;
- inability to enjoy things that used to bring pleasure;
- withdrawal from friends and family;
- irritability, anger, or anxiety;
- inability to concentrate;
- significant weight loss or gain;
- significant change in sleep patterns (inability to fall asleep, stay asleep, or get up in the morning);
- feelings of guilt or worthlessness;
- aches and pains (with no known medical cause);
- pessimism and indifference (not caring about anything in the present or future);
- thoughts of death or suicide.

When someone has five or more of these symptoms most of the time for two weeks or longer, that person is probably depressed.

Teens who are depressed may show other warning signs or symptoms, such as lack of interest or motivation, poor concentration, and low mental energy caused by depression. They also might have increased problems at school because of skipped classes.

Some teens with depression have other problems, too, and these can intensify feelings of worthlessness or inner pain. For example, people who cut themselves or who have eating disorders may have unrecognized depression that needs attention.

How Is Depression Different From Regular Sadness?

Everyone has some ups and downs, and sadness is a natural emotion. The normal stresses of life can lead anyone to feel sad every once in a while. Things like an argument with a friend, a breakup, doing poorly on a test, not being chosen for a team, or a best friend moving out of town can lead to feelings of sadness, hurt, disappointment, or grief. These reactions are usually brief and go away with a little time and care.

Depression is more than occasionally feeling blue, sad, or down in the dumps, though. Depression is a strong mood involving sadness, discouragement, despair, or hopelessness that lasts for weeks, months, or even longer. It interferes with a person's ability to participate in normal activities.

Depression affects a person's thoughts, outlook, and behavior as well as mood. In addition to a depressed mood, a person with depression can also feel tired, irritable, and notice changes in appetite.

When someone has depression, it can cloud everything. The world looks bleak and the person's thoughts reflect that hopelessness and helplessness. People with depression tend to have negative and self-critical thoughts. Sometimes, despite their true value, people with depression can feel worthless and unlovable.

Because of feelings of sadness and low energy, people with depression may pull away from those around them or from activities they once enjoyed. This usually makes them feel more lonely and isolated, making the depression and negative thinking worse.

Depression can be mild or severe. At its worst, depression can create such feelings of despair that a person thinks about suicide.

Depression can cause physical symptoms, too. Some people have an upset stomach, loss of appetite, weight gain or loss, headaches, and sleeping problems when they're depressed.

Getting Help

Depression is one of the most common emotional problems in the United States and around the world. The good news is that it's also one of the most treatable conditions. Therapists and other professionals can help. In fact, about 80 percent of people who get help for their depression have a better quality of life— they feel better and enjoy themselves in a way that they weren't able to before.

Treatment for depression can include talk therapy, medication, or a combination of both.

Talk therapy with a mental health professional is very effective in treating depression. Therapy sessions can help people understand more about why they feel depressed, and ways to combat it.

Sometimes, doctors prescribe medicine for a person who has depression. When prescribing medicine, a doctor will carefully monitor patients to make sure they get the right dose. The doctor will adjust the dose as necessary. It can take a few weeks before the person feels the medicine working. Because every person's brain is different, what works well for one person might not be good for another.

Everyone can benefit from mood-boosting activities like exercise, yoga, dance, journaling, or art. It can also help to keep busy no matter how tired you feel.

People who are depressed shouldn't wait and hope it will go away on its own because depression can be effectively treated. Friends or others need to step in if someone seems severely depressed and isn't getting help.

Many people find that it helps to open up to parents or other adults they trust. Simply saying, "I've been feeling really down lately and I think I'm depressed," can be a good way to begin the discussion. Ask your parent to arrange an appointment with a therapist. If a parent or family member can't help, turn to your school counselor, best friend, or a helpline to get help.

When Depression Is Severe

People who are extremely depressed and who may be thinking about hurting themselves or about suicide need help as soon as possible. When depression is this severe, it is a very real medical emergency, and an adult must be notified. Most communities have suicide hotlines where people can get guidance and support in an emergency.

Although it's important to be supportive, trying to cheer up a friend or reasoning with him or her probably won't work to help depression or suicidal feelings go away. Depression can be so strong that it outweighs a person's ability to respond to reason. Even if your friend has asked you to promise not to tell, severe depression is a situation where telling can save a life. The most important thing a depressed person can do is to get help. If you or a friend feels unsafe or out of control, get help now. Tell a trusted adult, call 911, or go to the emergency room.

☞ Remember!!

Depression doesn't mean a person is crazy. Depression (and the suffering that goes with it) is a real and recognized medical problem. Just as things can go wrong in all other organs of the body, things can go wrong in the most important organ of all: the brain. Luckily, most teens who get help for their depression go on to enjoy life and feel better about themselves.

Source: Copyright © 2007 The Nemours Foundation.

Chapter 9

How Is Depression Detected And Treated?

Depression, even the most severe cases, is a highly treatable disorder. As with many illnesses, the earlier that treatment can begin, the more effective it is and the greater the likelihood that recurrence can be prevented.

The first step to getting appropriate treatment is to visit a doctor. Certain medications, and some medical conditions such as viruses or a thyroid disorder, can cause the same symptoms as depression. A doctor can rule out these possibilities by conducting a physical examination, interview and lab tests. If the doctor can eliminate a medical condition as a cause, he or she should conduct a psychological evaluation or refer the patient to a mental health professional.

The doctor or mental health professional will conduct a complete diagnostic evaluation. He or she should discuss any family history of depression, and get a complete history of symptoms, for example, when they started, how long they have lasted, their severity, and whether they have occurred before and if so, how they were treated. He or she should also ask if the patient is using alcohol or drugs, and whether the patient is thinking about death or suicide.

About This Chapter: Text in this chapter is excerpted from "How is depression detected and treated?" National Institute of Mental Health, January 30, 2009. The complete text of this document, including references, is available online at http://www.nimh.nih.gov/health/publications/depression/how-is-depression-detected-and-treated.shtml.

Once diagnosed, a person with depression can be treated with a number of methods. The most common treatments are medication and psychotherapy.

Medication

Antidepressants work to normalize naturally occurring brain chemicals called neurotransmitters, notably serotonin and norepinephrine. Other antidepressants work on the neurotransmitter dopamine. Scientists studying depression have found that these particular chemicals are involved in regulating mood, but they are unsure of the exact ways in which they work.

The newest and most popular types of antidepressant medications are called selective serotonin reuptake inhibitors (SSRIs). SSRIs include fluoxetine (Prozac), citalopram (Celexa), sertraline (Zoloft) and several others. Serotonin and norepinephrine reuptake inhibitors (SNRIs) are similar to SSRIs and include venlafaxine (Effexor) and duloxetine (Cymbalta). SSRIs and SNRIs are more popular than the older classes of antidepressants, such as tricyclics—named for their chemical structure—and monoamine oxidase inhibitors (MAOIs) because they tend to have fewer side effects. However, medications affect everyone differently—no one-size-fits-all approach to medication exists. Therefore, for some people, tricyclics or MAOIs may be the best choice.

People taking MAOIs must adhere to significant food and medicinal restrictions to avoid potentially serious interactions. They must avoid certain foods that contain high levels of the chemical tyramine, which is found in many cheeses, wines and pickles, and some medications including decongestants. MAOIs interact with tyramine in such a way that may cause a sharp increase in blood pressure, which could lead to a stroke. A doctor should give a patient taking an MAOI a complete list of prohibited foods, medicines and substances.

For all classes of antidepressants, patients must take regular doses for at least three to four weeks before they are likely to experience a full therapeutic effect. They should continue taking the medication for the time specified by their doctor, even if they are feeling better, in order to prevent a relapse of the depression. Medication should be stopped only under a doctor's supervision. Some medications need to be gradually stopped to give the body time to adjust.

Although antidepressants are not habit–forming or addictive, abruptly ending an antidepressant can cause withdrawal symptoms or lead to a relapse. Some individuals, such as those with chronic or recurrent depression, may need to stay on the medication indefinitely.

In addition, if one medication does not work, patients should be open to trying another. Research funded by the National Institute of Mental Health (NIMH) has shown that patients who did not get well after taking a first medication increased their chances of becoming symptom-free after they switched to a different medication or added another medication to their existing one.

Sometimes stimulants, anti-anxiety medications, or other medications are used in conjunction with an antidepressant, especially if the patient has a co-existing mental or physical disorder. However, neither anti-anxiety medications nor stimulants are effective against depression when taken alone, and both should be taken only under a doctor's close supervision.

What Are The Side Effects Of Antidepressants?

Antidepressants may cause mild and often temporary side effects in some people, but they are usually not long-term. However, any unusual reactions or side effects that interfere with normal functioning should be reported to a doctor immediately.

The most common side effects associated with SSRIs and SNRIs include the following:

- **Headache:** Usually temporary and will subside.

- **Nausea:** Temporary and usually short-lived.

- **Insomnia And Nervousness** (trouble falling asleep or waking often during the night): May occur during the first few weeks but often subside over time or if the dose is reduced.

- **Agitation:** Feeling jittery.

- **Sexual Problems:** Both men and women can experience sexual problems including reduced sex drive, erectile dysfunction, delayed ejaculation, or inability to have an orgasm.

✤ It's A Fact!!
FDA Warning On Antidepressants

Despite the relative safety and popularity of selective serotonin reuptake inhibitors (SSRIs) and other antidepressants, some studies have suggested that they may have unintentional effects on some people, especially adolescents and young adults. In 2004, the Food and Drug Administration (FDA) conducted a thorough review of published and unpublished controlled clinical trials of antidepressants that involved nearly 4,400 children and adolescents. The review revealed that 4% of those taking antidepressants thought about or attempted suicide (although no suicides occurred), compared to 2% of those receiving placebos.

This information prompted the FDA, in 2005, to adopt a "black box" warning label on all antidepressant medications to alert the public about the potential increased risk of suicidal thinking or attempts in children and adolescents taking antidepressants. In 2007, the FDA proposed that makers of all antidepressant medications extend the warning to include young adults up through age 24. A "black box" warning is the most serious type of warning on prescription drug labeling.

The warning emphasizes that patients of all ages taking antidepressants should be closely monitored, especially during the initial weeks of treatment. Possible side effects to look for are worsening depression, suicidal thinking or behavior, or any unusual changes in behavior such as sleeplessness, agitation, or withdrawal from normal social situations. The warning adds that families and caregivers should also be told of the need for close monitoring and report any changes to the physician. The latest information from the FDA can be found on their website at www.fda.gov.

Results of a comprehensive review of pediatric trials conducted between 1988 and 2006 suggested that the benefits of antidepressant medications likely outweigh their risks to children and adolescents with major depression and anxiety disorders. The study was funded in part by the National Institute of Mental Health.

Also, the FDA issued a warning that combining an SSRI or SNRI antidepressant with one of the commonly-used "triptan" medications for migraine headache could cause a life-threatening "serotonin syndrome," marked by agitation, hallucinations, elevated body temperature, and rapid changes in blood pressure. Although most dramatic in the case of the MAOIs, newer antidepressants may also be associated with potentially dangerous interactions with other medications.

Source: National Institute of Mental Health, January 30, 2009.

Tricyclic antidepressants also can cause side effects such as these:

- **Dry Mouth:** It is helpful to drink plenty of water, chew gum, and clean teeth daily.

- **Constipation:** It is helpful to eat more bran cereals, prunes, fruits, and vegetables.

- **Bladder Problems:** Emptying the bladder may be difficult, and the urine stream may not be as strong as usual. Older men with enlarged prostate conditions may be more affected. The doctor should be notified if it is painful to urinate.

- **Sexual Problems:** Sexual functioning may change, and side effects are similar to those from SSRIs.

- **Blurred Vision:** Often passes soon and usually will not require a new corrective lenses prescription.

- **Drowsiness During The Day:** Usually passes soon, but driving or operating heavy machinery should be avoided while drowsiness occurs. The more sedating antidepressants are generally taken at bedtime to help sleep and minimize daytime drowsiness.

What About St. John's Wort?

The extract from St. John's wort (*Hypericum perforatum*), a bushy, wild-growing plant with yellow flowers, has been used for centuries in many folk and herbal remedies. Today in Europe, it is used extensively to treat mild to moderate depression. In the United States, it is one of the top-selling botanical products.

To address increasing American interests in St. John's wort, the National Institutes of Health conducted a clinical trial to determine the effectiveness of the herb in treating adults who have major depression. Involving 340 patients diagnosed with major depression, the eight-week trial randomly assigned one-third of them to a uniform dose of St. John's wort, one-third to a commonly prescribed SSRI, and one-third to a placebo. The trial found that St. John's wort was no more effective than the placebo in treating major depression. Another study is looking at the effectiveness of St. John's wort for treating mild or minor depression.

❖ It's A Fact!!

New Approach To Reducing
Suicide Attempts Among Depressed Teens

A novel treatment approach that includes medication plus a newly developed type of psychotherapy that targets suicidal thinking and behavior shows promise in treating depressed adolescents who had recently attempted suicide, according to a treatment development and pilot study funded by the National Institute of Mental Health (NIMH). The study, described in three articles, was published in the October 2009 issue of the *Journal of the American Academy of Child and Adolescent Psychiatry*.

Background: Youth who attempt suicide are particularly difficult to treat because they often leave treatment prematurely, and no specific interventions exist that reliably reduce suicidal thinking and behavior (suicidality). In addition, these teens often are excluded from clinical trials testing depression treatments. The Treatment of Adolescent Suicide Attempters Study (TASA) was developed to address this need and identify factors that may predict and mediate suicide reattempts among this vulnerable population. A novel psychotherapy used in the study—cognitive behavioral therapy for suicide prevention (CBT-SP—was developed to address the need for a specific psychotherapy that would prevent or reduce the risk for suicide reattempts among teens. CBT-SP consisted of a 12-week acute treatment phase focusing on safety planning, understanding the circumstances and vulnerabilities that lead to suicidal behavior, and building life skills to prevent a reattempt. A maintenance continuation phase followed the acute phase.

In the six-month, multisite pilot study, 124 adolescents who had recently attempted suicide were either randomized to or given the option of choosing one of three interventions—antidepressant medication only, CBT-SP only, or a combination of the two. Most participants preferred to choose their intervention, and most (93) chose combination therapy. Participants were assessed for suicidality at weeks six, 12, 18 and 24.

Results Of The Study: During the six-month treatment, 24 participants experienced a new suicidal event, defined as new onset or worsening of suicidal thinking or a suicide attempt. This rate of recurrence is lower than what previous studies among suicidal patients have found, suggesting that this treatment approach may be a promising intervention. In addition, more than 70 percent of these teens—a population that is typically difficult to keep in treatment—completed the acute phase of the therapy. However, many participants discontinued the treatment during the continuation phase, suggesting that treatment may need to include more frequent sessions during the acute phase, and limited sessions during the continuation phase.

The study revealed some characteristics that could predict recurrent suicidality, including high levels of self-reported suicidal thinking and depression, a history of abuse, two or more previous suicide attempts, and a strong sense of hopelessness. In addition, a high degree of family conflict predicted suicidality, while family support and cohesion acted as a protective factor against suicide reattempts. Other studies have found similar results, according to the researchers.

Significance: Although the study cannot address effectiveness of the treatment because it was not randomized, it sheds light on characteristics that identify who is most at risk for suicide reattempts, and what circumstances may help protect teens from attempting suicide again. In addition, the study found that 10 of the 24 suicide events occurred within four weeks of the beginning of the study—before they could receive adequate treatment. This suggests that a "front-loaded" intervention in which the most intense treatment is given early on, would likely reduce the risk of suicide reattempt even more.

What's Next: The effectiveness of CBT-SP—alone or in conjunction with antidepressant medication—will need to be tested in randomized clinical trials. In the meantime, because many suicide events occurred shortly after the beginning of the trial, the researchers suggest that clinicians emphasize safety planning and provide more intense therapy in the beginning of treatment. In addition, they note that therapy should focus on helping teens develop a tolerance for distress; work to improve the teen's home, school and social environment; and rigorously pursue coping strategies for teens who experienced childhood trauma such as abuse.

Source: "New Approach to Reducing Suicide Attempts Among Depressed Teens," a Science Update from the National Institute of Mental Health, September 29, 2009.

Other research has shown that St. John's wort can interact unfavorably with other medications, including those used to control HIV infection. On February 10, 2000, the FDA issued a Public Health Advisory letter stating that the herb appears to interfere with certain medications used to treat heart disease, depression, seizures, certain cancers, and organ transplant rejection. The herb also may interfere with the effectiveness of oral contraceptives. Because of these potential interactions, patients should always consult with their doctors before taking any herbal supplement.

Psychotherapy

Several types of psychotherapy—or "talk therapy"—can help people with depression.

Some regimens are short-term (10 to 20 weeks) and other regimens are longer-term, depending on the needs of the individual. Two main types of psychotherapies—cognitive-behavioral therapy (CBT) and interpersonal therapy (IPT)—have been shown to be effective in treating depression. By teaching new ways of thinking and behaving, CBT helps people change negative styles of thinking and behaving that may contribute to their depression. IPT helps people understand and work through troubled personal relationships that may cause their depression or make it worse.

For mild to moderate depression, psychotherapy may be the best treatment option. However, for major depression or for certain people, psychotherapy may not be enough. Studies have indicated that for adolescents, a combination of medication and psychotherapy may be the most effective approach to treating major depression and reducing the likelihood for recurrence. Similarly, a study examining depression treatment among older adults found that patients who responded to initial treatment of medication and IPT were less likely to have recurring depression if they continued their combination treatment for at least two years.

Electroconvulsive Therapy

For cases in which medication and/or psychotherapy does not help alleviate a person's treatment-resistant depression, electroconvulsive therapy (ECT) may be useful. ECT, formerly known as "shock therapy," once had a bad reputation. But in recent years, it has greatly improved and can provide relief for people with severe depression who have not been able to feel better with other treatments.

Before ECT is administered, a patient takes a muscle relaxant and is put under brief anesthesia. He or she does not consciously feel the electrical impulse administered in ECT. A patient typically will undergo ECT several times a week, and often will need to take an antidepressant or mood stabilizing medication to supplement the ECT treatments and prevent relapse. Although some patients will need only a few courses of ECT, others may need maintenance ECT, usually once a week at first, then gradually decreasing to monthly treatments for up to one year.

ECT may cause some short-term side effects, including confusion, disorientation and memory loss. But these side effects typically clear soon after treatment. Research has indicated that after one year of ECT treatments, patients showed no adverse cognitive effects.

What Efforts Are Underway To Improve Treatment?

Researchers are looking for ways to better understand, diagnose and treat depression among all groups of people. New potential treatments are being tested that give hope to those who live with depression that is particularly difficult to treat, and researchers are studying the risk factors for depression and how it affects the brain. NIMH continues to fund cutting-edge research into this debilitating disorder.

For more information on NIMH-funded research on depression, visit the NIMH website (www.nimh.nih.gov).

Chapter 10

Dealing With Teen Depression

The teenage years can be tough, and it's perfectly normal to feel sad or irritable every now and then. But if these feelings don't go away or become so intense that you can't handle them, you may be suffering from depression. The good news is that you don't have to feel this way. Help is available—all you have to do is ask. You also have more power over depression than you think. There are many things you can do to help yourself or a friend start feeling better.

What Depression Feels Like

If you think you are depressed, you're not alone. Depression is far more common in teens than you may think, and there is a lot of hope and help on the horizon. No matter what you believe, people love and care about you, and if you can muster the courage to talk about your depression, it can—and will—be resolved. Some people think that talking about sad feelings will make them worse, but the opposite is almost always true. It is very helpful to share your worries with someone who will listen and care, especially a trained professional who can guide you towards feeling better.

About This Chapter: "Dealing with Teen Depression," by Suzanne Barston, Melinda Smith, M.A., and Jeanne Segal, Ph.D., reprinted with permission from http://www.helpguide. org/mental/depression_teen_teenagers.htm. © 2009 Helpguide.org. All rights reserved. Helpguide provides a detailed list of related references for this article, including links to information from other websites. For a complete list of Helpguide's current resources related to depression in teens, including information about suicide and mental health, visit www.helpguide.org.

Signs And Symptoms Of Depression In Teens

It's hard to put into words how depression feels, and people experience it differently. There are, however, some common problems and symptoms that teens with depression experience.

- You constantly feel irritable, sad, or angry.

- Nothing seems fun anymore, and you just don't see the point of trying.

- You feel bad about yourself—worthless, guilty, or just "wrong" in some way.

- You sleep too much or not enough.

- You have frequent, unexplained headaches or other physical problems.

- Anything and everything makes you cry.

- You've gained or lost weight without consciously trying to.

- You just can't concentrate. Your grades may be plummeting because of it.

- You feel helpless and hopeless .

- You're thinking about death or suicide. (If this is true, talk to someone right away!)

✔ **Quick Tip**

Is your friend depressed?

If you're a teenager with a friend who seems down or troubled, you may suspect depression. But how do you know it's not just a passing phase or a bad mood? Look for common warning signs of teen depression:

- Your friend doesn't want to do the things you guys used to love to do.
- Your friend starts using alcohol or drugs or hanging with a bad crowd.
- Your friend stops going to classes and after school activities.
- Your friend talks about being bad, ugly, stupid, or worthless.
- Your friend starts talking about death or suicide.

Source: © 2009 Helpguide.org.

Dealing With Suicidal Thoughts

If your feelings become so overwhelming that you can't see any solution besides harming yourself or others, you need to get help right away. And yet, asking for help when you're in the midst of such strong emotions can be really tough. If talking to a stranger might be easier for you, call 800-273-TALK to speak in confidence to someone who can understand and help you deal with your feelings.

In the meantime, the following suggestions can help get you through until you feel ready to talk to someone:

- **There is ALWAYS another solution, even if you can't see it right now.** Many kids who have attempted suicide (and survived) say that they did it because they mistakenly felt there was no other solution to a problem they were experiencing. At the time, they could not see another way out—but in truth, they didn't really want to die. Remember that no matter how horribly you feel, these emotions will pass.

- **Having thoughts of hurting yourself or others does not make you a bad person.** Depression can make you think and feel things that are out of character. No one should judge you or condemn you for these feelings if you are brave enough to talk about them.

- **If your feelings are uncontrollable, tell yourself to wait 24 hours before you take any action.** This can give you time to really think things through and give yourself some distance from the strong emotions that are plaguing you. During this 24-hour period, try to talk to someone—anyone—as long as they are not another suicidal or depressed person. Call a hotline or talk to a friend. What do you have to lose?

If you're afraid you can't control yourself, make sure you are never alone. Even if you can't verbalize your feelings, just stay in public places, hang out with friends or family members, or go to a movie—anything to keep from being by yourself and in danger.

Above all, do not do anything that could result in permanent damage or death to yourself or others. Remember, suicide is a "permanent solution to a temporary problem." Help is available. All you need to do is take that first step and reach out.

What You Can Do To Feel Better

Depression is not your fault, and you didn't do anything to cause it. However, you do have some control over feeling better. Staying connected to friends and family, sharing your feelings with someone you trust, and making healthy lifestyle decisions can all have a hugely positive impact on your mood.

Ask for help if you're stressed. Stress and worry can take a big toll, even leading to depression. Talk to a teacher or school counselor if exams or classes seem overwhelming. Likewise, if you have a health concern you feel you can't talk to your parents about—such as a pregnancy scare or drug problem—seek medical attention at a clinic or see a doctor. A health professional can help you approach your parents (if that is required) and guide you toward appropriate treatment.

If you're dealing with relationship, friendship, or family problems, talk to an adult you trust. Your school may have a counselor you can go to for help, or you may want to ask your parents to make an appointment for you to see a therapist.

Try not to isolate yourself. When you're depressed, you may not feel like seeing anybody or doing anything. Just getting out of bed in the morning can be difficult, but isolating yourself only makes depression worse. Make it a point to stay social, even if that's the last thing you want to do. As you get out into the world, you may find yourself feeling better.

Spend time with friends, especially those who are active, upbeat, and make you feel good about yourself. Avoid hanging out with those who abuse drugs or alcohol, get you into trouble, or who make you feel insecure. It's also a good idea to limit the time you spend playing video games or surfing online.

Remember that you are not alone. You might be surprised at how many other teens suffer from depression. You are not alone, and neither is your depression a hopeless case. Even though it can feel like depression will never lift, it eventually will—and with proper treatment and healthy choices, that day can come even sooner. In the meantime, you might need therapy or medication to help you while you sort out your feelings. Look into your treatment options with your parents. If medication is being considered, do your research before making a decision, as some antidepressants used for adults can actually make teens feel worse.

Keep your body healthy. Making healthy lifestyle choices can do wonders for your mood. Things like diet and exercise have been shown to help depression. Ever heard of a "runners high"? You actually get a rush of endorphins from exercising, which makes you feel instantly happier. Physical activity can be as effective as medications or therapy for depression, so get involved in sports, ride your bike, or take a dance class. Any activity helps! Even a short walk can be beneficial.

As for food, it's true that you are what you eat. An improper diet can make you feel sluggish and tired, which worsens depression symptoms. Your body needs vitamins and minerals such as iron and the B vitamins. Make sure you're feeding your mind with plenty of fruits, vegetables, and whole grains. Talk to your parents, doctor or school nurse about how to ensure your diet is adequately nutritious.

✤ It's A Fact!!

There Are Benefits And Risks When Using Antidepressants

Antidepressants are used to treat depression and other illnesses. Depression and other illnesses can lead to suicide. In some children and teenagers, treatment with an antidepressant increases suicidal thinking or actions. It is important to discuss all the risks of treating depression and also the risks of not treating it. You should discuss all treatment choices with your healthcare provider, not just the use of antidepressants.

- Of all the antidepressants, only fluoxetine (Prozac™) has been FDA approved to treat pediatric depression.

- For obsessive compulsive disorder in children and teenagers, FDA has approved only fluoxetine (Prozac™), sertraline (Zoloft™), fluvoxamine, and clomipramine (Anafranil™).

Your healthcare provider may suggest other antidepressants based on your past experience or the past experience of other family members.

Source: Excerpted from "Medication Guide: About Using Antidepressants in Children and Teenagers," U.S. Food and Drug Administration (www.fda.gov), January 26, 2005.

Avoid alcohol and drugs. You may be tempted to drink or use drugs in an effort to escape from your feelings and get a "mood boost", even if just for a short time. However, substance use can not only make depression worse, but can cause you to become depressed in the first place. Alcohol and drug use can also increase suicidal feelings. In short, drinking and taking drugs will make you feel worse—not better—in the long run.

If you're addicted to alcohol or drugs, seek help. You will need special treatment for your substance problem on top of whatever treatment you're receiving for your depression.

Talking To Your Parents About Depression

As Will Smith once said, "parents just don't understand." Understatement of the year, huh? It may seem like there's no way your parents will be able to help, especially if they are always nagging you or getting angry about your behavior. The truth is, parents hate to see their kids hurting. They may feel frustrated because they don't understand what is going on with you or know how to help. Many parents don't know enough about depression to recognize it in their own kids. So, it may be up to you to educate them. You can refer them to the Helpguide website (www.helpguide .org), or look for further information online. Letting your parents know that you are feeling depressed will probably motivate them to get you the help you need.

If your parents are abusive in any way, or if they have problems of their own that makes it difficult for them to take care of you, find another adult you trust (such as a relative, teacher, counselor, or coach). This person can either help you approach your parents, or direct you toward the support you need. If you truly don't have anyone you can talk to, there are many hotlines, services, and support groups that can help. Visit the Helpguide website for a list of resources, call 800-273-TALK

✔ Quick Tip

If you are suffering and don't know where to turn...

Call the Nineline's 24-hour hotline for children and teens at 800-999-9999. It's free, confidential, and always available, so call if you need to talk to somebody or want information on where to get help in your area.

Source: © 2009 Helpguide.org.

if you need to talk to someone about suicidal thoughts, or 800-999-9999 for help dealing with a crisis. No matter what, talk to someone, especially if you are having any thoughts of harming yourself or others. Asking for help is the bravest thing you can do, and the first step on your way to feeling better.

Helping A Depressed Friend

Depressed teens typically rely on their friends more than their parents or other adults in their lives, so you may find yourself in the position of being the first—or only—person that they talk to about their feelings. While this might seem like a huge responsibility, there are many things you can do to help.

- **Get your friend to talk to you.** Starting a conversation about depression can be daunting, but you can say something simple: "You seem like you are really down, and not yourself. I really want to help you. Is there anything I can do?"

- **Know that your friend doesn't expect you to have the answers.** Your friend probably just needs someone to listen and be supportive. By listening and responding in a non-judgmental and reassuring manner, you are helping in a major way.

- **Encourage your friend to get help.** Urge your depressed friend to talk to a parent, teacher, or counselor. It might be scary for your friend to admit to an authority figure that there is a problem. Having you there might help, so offer to go along for support.

- **Stick with your friend through the hard times.** Depression can make people do and say things that are hurtful or strange. But your friend is going through a very difficult time, so try not to take it personally. Once your friend gets help, he or she will go back to being the person you know and love. In the meantime, make sure you have other friends or family taking care of you—your feelings are important and need to be respected, too.

- **Speak up if your friend is suicidal.** If your friend is joking or talking about suicide, giving possessions away, or saying goodbye, tell a trusted adult immediately. Your only responsibility at this point is to get your friend help, and get it fast. Even if you promised not to tell, your friend needs your help. It's better to have a friend who is temporarily angry at you than one who is no longer alive.

Chapter 11

Bipolar Disorder

Recently, doctors have been diagnosing more children with bipolar disorder, sometimes called manic-depressive illness. But what does this illness really mean for a young person?

Bipolar disorder, also known as manic-depressive illness, is a brain disorder that causes unusual shifts in mood and energy. It can also make it hard for someone to carry out day-to-day tasks, such as going to school or hanging out with friends. Symptoms of bipolar disorder are severe. They are different from the normal ups and downs that everyone goes through from time to time. They can result in damaged relationships, poor school performance, and even suicide. But bipolar disorder can be treated, and people with this illness can lead full and productive lives.

Bipolar disorder often develops in a person's late teens or early adult years, but some people have their first symptoms during childhood. At least half of all cases start before age 25.

Common Symptoms Of Bipolar Disorder In Children And Teens

Youth with bipolar disorder experience unusually intense emotional states that occur in distinct periods called "mood episodes." An overly joyful or over-excited state is called a manic episode, and an extremely sad or hopeless state

About This Chapter: The text in this chapter is excerpted and adapted from "Bipolar Disorder in Children and Teens: A Parent's Guide," National Institute of Mental Health, 2008.

is called a depressive episode. Sometimes, a mood episode includes symptoms of both mania and depression. This is called a mixed state. People with bipolar disorder also may be explosive and irritable during a mood episode.

Extreme changes in energy, activity, sleep, and behavior go along with these changes in mood.

Symptoms Of Mania: Mood Changes

- Being in an overly silly or joyful mood that's unusual; different from times when a child might usually get silly and have fun

- Having an extremely short temper; an irritable mood that is unusual

Symptoms Of Mania: Behavioral Changes

- Sleeping little but not feeling tired

- Talking a lot and having racing thoughts

- Having trouble concentrating, attention jumping from one thing to the next in an unusual way

- Talking and thinking about sex more often

- Behaving in risky ways more often, seeking pleasure a lot, and doing more activities than usual

Symptoms Of Depression: Mood Changes

- Being in a sad mood that lasts a long time

- Losing interest in activities they once enjoyed

- Feeling worthless or guilty

Symptoms Of Depression: Behavioral Changes

- Complaining about pain more often, such as headaches, stomach aches, and muscle pains

- Eating a lot more or less and gaining or losing a lot of weight

- Sleeping or oversleeping when these were not problems before

- Losing energy

- Recurring thoughts of death or suicide

It's normal for almost every child or teen to have some of these symptoms sometimes. These passing changes should not be confused with bipolar disorder.

Symptoms of bipolar disorder are not like the normal changes in mood and energy that everyone has now and then. Bipolar symptoms are more extreme and tend to last for most of the day, nearly every day, for at least one week. Also, depressive or manic episodes include moods very different from a child's normal mood, and the behaviors described above may start at the same time. Sometimes the symptoms of bipolar disorder are so severe that the child needs to be treated in a hospital.

In addition to mania and depression, bipolar disorder can cause a range of moods. On the depression side, the range includes severe depression, moderate depression, and mild low mood. Moderate depression may cause less extreme symptoms, and mild low mood is called dysthymia when it is chronic or long-term. In the middle of the scale is normal or balanced mood.

Sometimes, a child may have more energy and be more active than normal, but not show the severe signs of a full-blown manic episode. When this happens, it is called hypomania, and it generally lasts for at least four days in a row. Hypomania causes noticeable changes in behavior, but does not harm a child's ability to function in the way mania does.

❖ **It's A Fact!!**

Watch out for any sign of suicidal thinking or behaviors. Take these signs seriously. On average, people with early-onset bipolar disorder have greater risk for attempting suicide than those whose symptoms start in adulthood. One large study on bipolar disorder in children and teens found that more than one-third of study participants made at least one serious suicide attempt. Some suicide attempts are carefully planned and others are not. Either way, it is important to understand that suicidal feelings and actions are symptoms of an illness that must be treated.

Bipolar Disorder Affects Children And Teens Differently Than Adults

Bipolar disorder that starts during childhood or during the teen years is called early-onset bipolar disorder. Early-onset bipolar disorder seems to be more severe than the forms that first appear in older teens and adults. Youth with bipolar disorder are different from adults with bipolar disorder. Young people with the illness appear to have more frequent mood switches, are sick more often, and have more mixed episodes.

Other Illnesses Often Co-exist With Bipolar Disorder In Children And Teens

Several illnesses may develop in people with bipolar disorder.

Alcoholism: Adults with bipolar disorder are at very high risk of developing a substance abuse problem. Young people with bipolar disorder may have the same risk.

ADHD: Many children with bipolar disorder have a history of attention deficit hyperactivity disorder (ADHD). One study showed that ADHD is more common in people whose bipolar disorder started during childhood, compared with people whose bipolar disorder started later in life. Children who have co-occurring ADHD and bipolar disorder may have difficulty concentrating and controlling their activity. This may happen even when they are not manic or depressed.

Anxiety Disorders: Anxiety disorders, such as separation anxiety and generalized anxiety disorder, also commonly co-occur with bipolar disorder. This may happen in both children and adults. Children who have both types of disorders tend to develop bipolar disorder at a younger age and have more hospital stays related to mental illness.

Other Mental Disorders: Some mental disorders cause symptoms similar to bipolar disorder. Two examples are major depression (sometimes called unipolar depression) and ADHD. If you look at symptoms only, there is no way to tell the difference between major depression and a depressive episode in bipolar disorder. For this reason, be sure to tell a diagnosing doctor of any past manic symptoms or episodes that may have been experienced. In contrast, ADHD does not have episodes. ADHD symptoms may resemble mania in some ways, but they tend to be more constant than in a manic episode of bipolar disorder.

Treatments Available For Children And Teens With Bipolar Disorder

To date, there is no cure for bipolar disorder. However, treatment with medications, psychotherapy (talk therapy), or both may help people get better.

It's important for you to know that young people sometimes respond differently to psychiatric medications than adults do.

To treat children and teens with bipolar disorder, doctors often rely on information about treating adults. This is because there haven't been many studies on treating young people with the illness, although several have been started recently.

Medications

Before starting medication, the doctor will want to determine the patient's physical and mental health. This is called a "baseline" assessment. The patient will need regular follow-up visits to monitor treatment progress and side effects. Most children with bipolar disorder will also need long-term or even lifelong medication treatment. This is often the best way to manage symptoms and prevent relapse, or a return of symptoms.

It's better to limit the number and dose of medications. A good way to remember this is "start low, go slow." Talk to the psychiatrist about using the smallest amount of medication that helps relieve symptoms. To judge a medication's effectiveness, the patient may need to take a medication for several weeks or months. The doctor needs this time to decide whether to switch to a different medication. Because children's symptoms are complex, it's not unusual for them to need more than one type of medication.

Keep a daily log of the most troublesome symptoms. Doing so can make it easier for you and the doctor to decide whether a medication is helpful. Also, be sure to tell the psychiatrist about all other prescription drugs, over-the-counter medications, or natural supplements you are taking. Taking certain medications and supplements together may cause unwanted or dangerous effects.

Psychotherapy

In addition to medication, psychotherapy ("talk" therapy) can be an effective treatment for bipolar disorder. Studies in adults show that it can provide support, education, and guidance to people with bipolar disorder and their families. Psychotherapy may also help children keep taking their medications to stay healthy and prevent relapse.

Children and teens may also benefit from therapies that address problems at school, work, or in the community.

Some psychotherapy treatments used for bipolar disorder include the following:

- Cognitive behavioral therapy helps young people with bipolar disorder learn to change harmful or negative thought patterns and behaviors.

- Family-focused therapy includes a child's family members. It helps enhance family coping strategies, such as recognizing new episodes early and helping their child.

- This therapy also improves communication and problem-solving.

- Interpersonal and social rhythm therapy helps children and teens with bipolar disorder improve their relationships with others and manage their daily routines. Regular daily routines and sleep schedules may help protect against manic episodes.

- Psychoeducation teaches young people with bipolar disorder about the illness and its treatment. This treatment helps people recognize signs of relapse so they can seek treatment early, before a full-blown episode occurs. Psychoeducation also may be helpful for family members and caregivers.

Other types of therapies may be tried as well, or used along with those mentioned above. The number, frequency, and type of psychotherapy sessions should be based on the patient's treatment needs.

A licensed psychologist, social worker, or counselor typically provides these therapies. This professional often works with a child's psychiatrist to monitor care. Some may also be licensed to prescribe medications; check the laws in your state.

In addition to getting therapy to reduce symptoms of bipolar disorder, children and teens may also benefit from therapies that address problems at school, work, or in the community. Such therapies may target communication skills, problem-solving skills, or skills for school or work. Other programs, such as those provided by social welfare programs or support and advocacy groups, can help as well.

Some children with bipolar disorder may also have learning disorders or language problems. The patient's school may need to make accommodations that reduce the stresses of a school day and provide proper support or interventions.

Families Of Children With Bipolar Disorder Can Get Help

As with other serious illnesses, taking care of a child with bipolar disorder is incredibly hard on the parents, family, and other caregivers. Caregivers often must tend to the medical needs of their child while dealing with how it affects their own health. The stress that caregivers are under may lead to missed work or lost free time. It can strain relationships with people who do not understand the situation and lead to physical and mental exhaustion.

❖ It's A Fact!!

There is no cure for bipolar disorder, but it can be treated effectively over the long term. Doctors and families of children with bipolar disorder should keep track of symptoms and treatment effects to decide whether changes to the treatment plan are needed.

If the patient has other psychiatric illnesses, such as an anxiety disorder, eating disorder, or substance abuse disorder, he or she may be more likely to experience a relapse—especially depressive symptoms. Scientists are unsure how these co-existing illnesses increase the chance of relapse.

Working closely with a doctor and a therapist and talking openly about treatment choices can make treatment more effective. You may need to talk about changing the treatment plan occasionally to help manage the illness most effectively.

Also, you may wish to keep a chart of daily mood symptoms, treatments, sleep patterns, and life events, which can help you better understand the illness. Sometimes this is called a mood chart or a daily life chart. It can help the doctor track and treat the illness more effectively.

Stress from caregiving can make it hard to cope with a child's bipolar symptoms. One study shows that if a caregiver is under a lot of stress, his or her loved one has more trouble sticking to the treatment plan, which increases the chance for a major bipolar episode. It is important for parents to take care of their own physical and mental health. They may also find it helpful to join a local support group or an online support group.

Finding Help

If you are unsure where to go for help, ask your family doctor. Others who can help are listed below:

- Mental health specialists, such as psychiatrists, psychologists, social workers, or mental health counselors

- Health maintenance organizations

- Community mental health centers

- Hospital psychiatry departments and outpatient clinics

- Mental health programs at universities or medical schools

- State hospital outpatient clinics

- Family services, social agencies, or clergy

- Peer support groups

- Private clinics and facilities

- Employee assistance programs

- Local medical and/or psychiatric societies

> ✔ Quick Tip
> **What To Do
> In A Crisis**
>
> - Call your doctor.
>
> - Call 911 or go to a hospital emergency room to get immediate help or ask a friend or family member to help you do these things.
>
> - Call the toll-free, 24-hour hotline of the National Suicide Prevention Lifeline at 1-800-273-TALK (1-800-273-8255); TTY: 1-800-799-4TTY (4889) to talk to a trained counselor.
>
> - Make sure you are not left alone.

You can also check the phone book under "mental health," "health," "social services," "hotlines," or "physicians" for phone numbers and addresses. An emergency room doctor can also provide temporary help and can tell you where and how to get further help.

Chapter 12

Anxiety Disorders

Anxiety disorders cause people to be filled with fearfulness and uncertainty. Unlike the relatively mild, brief anxiety caused by a stressful event (such as speaking in public or a first date), anxiety disorders last at least six months and can get worse if they are not treated. Anxiety disorders commonly occur along with other mental or physical illnesses, including alcohol or substance abuse, which may mask anxiety symptoms or make them worse. In some cases, these other illnesses need to be treated before a person will respond to treatment for the anxiety disorder.

Effective therapies for anxiety disorders are available, and research is uncovering new treatments that can help most people with anxiety disorders lead productive, fulfilling lives. If you think you have an anxiety disorder, you should seek information and treatment right away.

Panic Disorder

Panic disorder is a real illness that can be successfully treated. It is characterized by sudden attacks of terror, usually accompanied by a pounding heart, sweatiness, weakness, faintness, or dizziness. During these attacks, people with panic disorder may flush or feel chilled; their hands may tingle or feel numb; and they may experience nausea, chest pain, or smothering sensations. Panic attacks usually produce a sense of unreality, a fear of impending doom, or a fear of losing control.

About This Chapter: Text in this chapter is excerpted from "Anxiety Disorders," National Institute of Mental Health (www.nimh.nih.gov), September 2009.

A fear of one's own unexplained physical symptoms is also a symptom of panic disorder. People having panic attacks sometimes believe they are having heart attacks, losing their minds, or on the verge of death. They can't predict when or where an attack will occur, and between episodes many worry intensely and dread the next attack.

Panic attacks can occur at any time, even during sleep. An attack usually peaks within 10 minutes, but some symptoms may last much longer.

Panic disorder is twice as common in women as men. Panic attacks often begin in late adolescence or early adulthood, but not everyone who experiences panic attacks will develop panic disorder. Many people have just one attack and never have another. The tendency to develop panic attacks appears to be inherited.

People who have full-blown, repeated panic attacks can become very disabled by their condition and should seek treatment before they start to avoid places or situations where panic attacks have occurred. For example, if a panic attack happened in an elevator, someone with panic disorder may develop a fear of elevators that could affect the choice of a job or an apartment, and restrict where that person can seek medical attention or enjoy entertainment.

Some people's lives become so restricted that they avoid normal activities, such as grocery shopping or driving. About one-third become housebound or are able to confront a feared situation only when accompanied by a spouse or other trusted person. When the condition progresses this far, it is called agoraphobia, or fear of open spaces.

Early treatment can often prevent agoraphobia, but people with panic disorder may sometimes go from doctor to doctor for years and visit the emergency room repeatedly before someone correctly diagnoses their condition. This is unfortunate, because panic disorder is one of the most treatable of all the anxiety disorders, responding in most cases to certain kinds of medication or certain kinds of cognitive psychotherapy, which help change thinking patterns that lead to fear and anxiety.

Panic disorder is often accompanied by other serious problems, such as depression, drug abuse, or alcoholism. These conditions need to be treated separately. Symptoms of depression include feelings of sadness or hopelessness, changes in appetite or sleep patterns, low energy, and difficulty concentrating. Most people with depression can be effectively treated with antidepressant medications, certain types of psychotherapy, or a combination of the two.

Obsessive-Compulsive Disorder

People with obsessive-compulsive disorder (OCD) have persistent, upsetting thoughts (obsessions) and use rituals (compulsions) to control the anxiety these thoughts produce. Most of the time, the rituals end up controlling them.

For example, if people are obsessed with germs or dirt, they may develop a compulsion to wash their hands over and over again. If they develop an obsession with intruders, they may lock and relock their doors many times before going to bed. Being afraid of social embarrassment may prompt people with OCD to comb their hair compulsively in front of a mirror-sometimes they get "caught" in the mirror and can't move away from it. Performing such rituals is not pleasurable. At best, it produces temporary relief from the anxiety created by obsessive thoughts.

Other common rituals are a need to repeatedly check things, touch things (especially in a particular sequence), or count things. Some common obsessions include having frequent thoughts of violence and harming loved ones, persistently thinking about performing sexual acts the person dislikes, or having thoughts that are prohibited by religious beliefs. People with OCD may also be preoccupied with order and symmetry, have difficulty throwing things out (so they accumulate), or hoard unneeded items.

Healthy people also have rituals, such as checking to see if the stove is off several times before leaving the house. The difference is that people with OCD perform their rituals even though doing so interferes with daily life and they find the repetition distressing. Although most adults with OCD recognize that what they are doing is senseless, some adults and most children may not realize that their behavior is out of the ordinary.

OCD can be accompanied by eating disorders, other anxiety disorders, or depression. It strikes men and women in roughly equal numbers and usually appears in childhood, adolescence, or early adulthood. One-third of adults with OCD develop symptoms as children, and research indicates that OCD might run in families.

The course of the disease is quite varied. Symptoms may come and go, ease over time, or get worse. If OCD becomes severe, it can keep a person from working or carrying out normal responsibilities at home. People with OCD may try to help themselves by avoiding situations that trigger their obsessions, or they may use alcohol or drugs to calm themselves.

OCD usually responds well to treatment with certain medications and/ or exposure-based psychotherapy, in which people face situations that cause fear or anxiety and become less sensitive (desensitized) to them. The National Institute of Mental Health (NIMH) is supporting research into new treatment approaches for people whose OCD does not respond well to the usual therapies. These approaches include combination and augmentation (add-on) treatments, as well as modern techniques such as deep brain stimulation.

Post-Traumatic Stress Disorder

Post-traumatic stress disorder (PTSD) develops after a terrifying ordeal that involved physical harm or the threat of physical harm. The person who develops PTSD may have been the one who was harmed, the harm may have happened to a loved one, or the person may have witnessed a harmful event that happened to loved ones or strangers.

PTSD was first brought to public attention in relation to war veterans, but it can result from a variety of traumatic incidents, such as mugging, rape, torture, being kidnapped or held captive, child abuse, car accidents, train wrecks, plane crashes, bombings, or natural disasters such as floods or earthquakes.

People with PTSD may startle easily, become emotionally numb (especially in relation to people with whom they used to be close), lose interest in things they used to enjoy, have trouble feeling affectionate, be irritable, become more aggressive, or even become violent. They avoid situations that remind them of the original incident, and anniversaries of the incident are often very difficult. PTSD symptoms seem to be worse if the event that triggered them was deliberately initiated by another person, as in a mugging or a kidnapping.

Most people with PTSD repeatedly relive the trauma in their thoughts during the day and in nightmares when they sleep. These are called flashbacks. Flashbacks may consist of images, sounds, smells, or feelings, and are often triggered by ordinary occurrences, such as a door slamming or a car backfiring on the street. A person having a flashback may lose touch with reality and believe that the traumatic incident is happening all over again.

Not every traumatized person develops full-blown or even minor PTSD. Symptoms usually begin within three months of the incident but occasionally emerge years afterward. They must last more than a month to be considered PTSD. The course of the illness varies. Some people recover within six months, while others have symptoms that last much longer. In some people, the condition becomes chronic.

PTSD can occur at any age, including childhood. Women are more likely to develop PTSD than men, and there is some evidence that susceptibility to the disorder may run in families. PTSD is often accompanied by depression, substance abuse, or one or more of the other anxiety disorders.

Certain kinds of medication and certain kinds of psychotherapy usually treat the symptoms of PTSD very effectively.

Social Phobia (Social Anxiety Disorder)

Social phobia, also called social anxiety disorder, is diagnosed when people become overwhelmingly anxious and excessively self-conscious in everyday social situations. People with social phobia have an intense, persistent, and chronic fear of being watched and judged by others and of doing things that will embarrass them. They can worry for days or weeks before a dreaded situation. This fear may become so severe that it interferes with work, school, and other ordinary activities, and can make it hard to make and keep friends.

While many people with social phobia realize that their fears about being with people are excessive or unreasonable, they are unable to overcome them. Even if they manage to confront their fears and be around others, they are usually very anxious beforehand, are intensely uncomfortable throughout the encounter, and worry about how they were judged for hours afterward.

Social phobia can be limited to one situation (such as talking to people, eating or drinking, or writing on a blackboard in front of others) or may be so broad (such as in generalized social phobia) that the person experiences anxiety around almost anyone other than the family.

Physical symptoms that often accompany social phobia include blushing, profuse sweating, trembling, nausea, and difficulty talking. When these symptoms occur, people with social phobia feel as though all eyes are focused on them.

Women and men are equally likely to develop social phobia, which usually begins in childhood or early adolescence. There is some evidence that genetic factors are involved. Social phobia is often accompanied by other anxiety disorders or depression, and substance abuse may develop if people try to self-medicate their anxiety.

Social phobia can be successfully treated with certain kinds of psychotherapy or medications.

✿ It's A Fact!!
Treatment Of PTSD

Today, there are good treatments available for post-traumatic stress disorder (PTSD). When you have PTSD dealing with the past can be hard. Instead of telling others how you feel, you may keep your feelings bottled up. But talking with a therapist can help you get better.

Cognitive-behavioral therapy (CBT) is one type of counseling. It appears to be the most effective type of counseling for PTSD. There are different types of cognitive behavioral therapies such as cognitive therapy and exposure therapy. The U.S. Department of Veterans Affairs (VA) is providing two forms of cognitive-behavioral therapy to veterans with PTSD: cognitive processing therapy (CPT) and prolonged exposure therapy (PE). There is also a similar kind of therapy called eye movement desensitization and reprocessing (EMDR) that is used for PTSD. Medications have also been shown to be effective. A type of drug known as a selective serotonin reuptake inhibitor (SSRI), which is also used for depression, is effective for PTSD.

Source: From "Treatment of PTSD," U.S. Department of Veterans Affairs, (www.ptsd .va.gov), November 2009.

Specific Phobias

A specific phobia is an intense, irrational fear of something that poses little or no actual danger. Some of the more common specific phobias are centered around closed-in places, heights, escalators, tunnels, highway driving, water, flying, dogs, and injuries involving blood. Such phobias aren't just extreme fear; they are irrational fear of a particular thing. You may be able to ski the world's tallest mountains with ease but be unable to go above the 5th floor of an office building. While adults with phobias realize that these fears are irrational, they often find that facing, or even thinking about facing, the feared object or situation brings on a panic attack or severe anxiety.

Specific phobias are twice as common in women as men. They usually appear in childhood or adolescence and tend to persist into adulthood. The causes of specific phobias are not well understood, but there is some evidence that the tendency to develop them may run in families. Specific phobias respond very well to carefully targeted psychotherapy.

Generalized Anxiety Disorder

People with generalized anxiety disorder (GAD) go through the day filled with exaggerated worry and tension, even though there is little or nothing to provoke it. They anticipate disaster and are overly concerned about health issues, money, family problems, or difficulties at work. Sometimes just the thought of getting through the day produces anxiety.

GAD is diagnosed when a person worries excessively about a variety of everyday problems for at least six months. People with GAD can't seem to get rid of their concerns, even though they usually realize that their anxiety is more intense than the situation warrants. They can't relax, startle easily, and have difficulty concentrating. Often they have trouble falling asleep or staying asleep. Physical symptoms that often accompany the anxiety include fatigue, headaches, muscle tension, muscle aches, difficulty swallowing, trembling, twitching, irritability, sweating, nausea, lightheadedness, having to go to the bathroom frequently, feeling out of breath, and hot flashes.

When their anxiety level is mild, people with GAD can function socially and hold down a job. Although they don't avoid certain situations as a result of their disorder, people with GAD can have difficulty carrying out the simplest daily activities if their anxiety is severe.

GAD affects twice as many women as men. The disorder develops gradually and can begin at any point in the life cycle, although the years of highest risk are between childhood and middle age. There is evidence that genes play a modest role in GAD.

Other anxiety disorders, depression, or substance abuse often accompany GAD, which rarely occurs alone. GAD is commonly treated with medication or cognitive-behavioral therapy, but co-occurring conditions must also be treated using the appropriate therapies.

Treatment Of Anxiety Disorders

In general, anxiety disorders are treated with medication, specific types of psychotherapy, or both. Treatment choices depend on the problem and the person's preference. Before treatment begins, a doctor must conduct a careful diagnostic evaluation to determine whether a person's symptoms are caused by an anxiety disorder or a physical problem. If an anxiety disorder is diagnosed, the type of disorder or the combination of disorders that are present must be identified, as well as any coexisting conditions, such as depression or substance abuse. Sometimes alcoholism, depression, or other coexisting conditions have such a strong effect on the individual that treating the anxiety disorder must wait until the coexisting conditions are brought under control.

People with anxiety disorders who have already received treatment should tell their current doctor about that treatment in detail. If they received medication, they should tell their doctor what medication was used, what the dosage was at the beginning of treatment, whether the dosage was increased or decreased while they were under treatment, what side effects occurred, and whether the treatment helped them become less anxious. If they received psychotherapy, they should describe the type of therapy, how often they attended sessions, and whether the therapy was useful.

Often people believe that they have "failed" at treatment or that the treatment didn't work for them when, in fact, it was not given for an adequate length of time or was administered incorrectly. Sometimes people must try several different treatments or combinations of treatment before they find the one that works for them.

Medication

Medication will not cure anxiety disorders, but it can keep them under control while the person receives psychotherapy. Medication must be prescribed by physicians, usually psychiatrists, who can either offer psychotherapy themselves or work as a team with psychologists, social workers, or counselors who provide psychotherapy. The principal medications used for anxiety disorders are antidepressants, anti-anxiety drugs, and beta-blockers to control some of the physical symptoms. With proper treatment, many people with anxiety disorders can lead normal, fulfilling lives.

Antidepressants: Antidepressants were developed to treat depression but are also effective for anxiety disorders. Although these medications begin to alter brain chemistry after the very first dose, their full effect requires a series of changes to occur; it is usually about four to six weeks before symptoms start to fade. It is important to continue taking these medications long enough to let them work.

SSRIs: Some of the newest antidepressants are called selective serotonin reuptake inhibitors, or SSRIs. SSRIs alter the levels of the neurotransmitter serotonin in the brain, which, like other neurotransmitters, helps brain cells communicate with one another.

Fluoxetine (Prozac®), sertraline (Zoloft®), escitalopram (Lexapro®), paroxetine (Paxil®), and citalopram (Celexa®) are some of the SSRIs commonly prescribed for panic disorder, OCD, PTSD, and social phobia. SSRIs are also used to treat panic disorder when it occurs in combination with OCD, social phobia, or depression. Venlafaxine (Effexor®), a drug closely related to the SSRIs, is used to treat GAD. These medications are started at low doses and gradually increased until they have a beneficial effect.

SSRIs have fewer side effects than older antidepressants, but they sometimes produce slight nausea or jitters when people first start to take them. These symptoms fade with time. Some people also experience sexual dysfunction with SSRIs, which may be helped by adjusting the dosage or switching to another SSRI.

Tricyclics: Tricyclics are older than SSRIs and work as well as SSRIs for anxiety disorders other than OCD. They are also started at low doses that are gradually increased. They sometimes cause dizziness, drowsiness, dry mouth, and weight gain, which can usually be corrected by changing the dosage or switching to another tricyclic medication.

Tricyclics include imipramine (Tofranil®), which is prescribed for panic disorder and GAD, and clomipramine (Anafranil®), which is the only tricyclic antidepressant useful for treating OCD.

MAOIs: Monoamine oxidase inhibitors (MAOIs) are the oldest class of antidepressant medications. The MAOIs most commonly prescribed for anxiety disorders are phenelzine (Nardil®), followed by tranylcypromine (Parnate®), and isocarboxazid (Marplan®), which are useful in treating panic

---

✣ It's A Fact!!

Selective serotonin reuptake inhibitors (SSRIs) are a type of antidepressant medicine. These can help you feel less sad and worried. They appear to be helpful, and for some people they are very effective. SSRIs include citalopram (Celexa), fluoxetine (such as Prozac), paroxetine (Paxil), and sertraline (Zoloft).

Chemicals in your brain affect the way you feel. When you have or depression you may not have enough of a chemical called serotonin. SSRIs raise the level of serotonin in your brain.

There are other medications that have been used with some success. Talk to your doctor about which medications are right for you.

Source: From "Treatment of PTSD," U.S. Department of Veterans Affairs, (www.ptsd.va.gov), November 2009.

disorder and social phobia. People who take MAOIs cannot eat a variety of foods and beverages (including cheese and red wine) that contain tyramine or take certain medications, including some types of birth control pills, pain relievers (such as Advil®, Motrin®, or Tylenol®), cold and allergy medications, and herbal supplements; these substances can interact with MAOIs to cause dangerous increases in blood pressure. The development of a new MAOI skin patch may help lessen these risks. MAOIs can also react with SSRIs to produce a serious condition called "serotonin syndrome," which can cause confusion, hallucinations, increased sweating, muscle stiffness, seizures, changes in blood pressure or heart rhythm, and other potentially life-threatening conditions.

Anti-Anxiety Drugs: High-potency benzodiazepines combat anxiety and have few side effects other than drowsiness. Because people can get used to them and may need higher and higher doses to get the same effect, benzodiazepines are generally prescribed for short periods of time, especially for people who have abused drugs or alcohol and who become dependent on medication easily. One exception to this rule is people with panic disorder, who can take benzodiazepines for up to a year without harm.

Clonazepam (Klonopin®) is used for social phobia and GAD, lorazepam (Ativan®) is helpful for panic disorder, and alprazolam (Xanax®) is useful for both panic disorder and GAD.

Some people experience withdrawal symptoms if they stop taking benzo-diazepines abruptly instead of tapering off, and anxiety can return once the medication is stopped. These potential problems have led some physicians to shy away from using these drugs or to use them in inadequate doses.

Buspirone (BuSpar®), an azapirone, is a newer anti-anxiety medication used to treat GAD. Possible side effects include dizziness, headaches, and nausea. Unlike benzodiazepines, buspirone must be taken consistently for at least two weeks to achieve an anti-anxiety effect.

Beta-Blockers: Beta-blockers, such as propranolol (Inderal®), which is used to treat heart conditions, can prevent the physical symptoms that accompany certain anxiety disorders, particularly social phobia. When a feared situation can be predicted (such as giving a speech), a doctor may prescribe a beta-blocker to keep physical symptoms of anxiety under control.

Psychotherapy

Psychotherapy involves talking with a trained mental health professional, such as a psychiatrist, psychologist, social worker, or counselor, to discover what caused an anxiety disorder and how to deal with its symptoms.

Cognitive-Behavioral Therapy

Cognitive-behavioral therapy (CBT) is very useful in treating anxiety disorders. The cognitive part helps people change the thinking patterns that support their fears, and the behavioral part helps people change the way they react to anxiety-provoking situations.

For example, CBT can help people with panic disorder learn that their panic attacks are not really heart attacks and help people with social phobia learn how to overcome the belief that others are always watching and judging them. When people are ready to confront their fears, they are shown how to use exposure techniques to desensitize themselves to situations that trigger their anxieties.

People with OCD who fear dirt and germs are encouraged to get their hands dirty and wait increasing amounts of time before washing them. The therapist helps the person cope with the anxiety that waiting produces; after the exercise has been repeated a number of times, the anxiety diminishes. People with social phobia may be encouraged to spend time in feared social situations without giving in to the temptation to flee and to make small social blunders and observe how people

> **✔ Quick Tip**
> **Taking Medications**
>
> Before taking medication for an anxiety disorder:
>
> • Ask your doctor to tell you about the effects and side effects of the drug.
>
> • Tell your doctor about any alternative therapies or over-the-counter medications you are using.
>
> • Ask your doctor when and how the medication should be stopped. Some drugs can't be stopped abruptly but must be tapered off slowly under a doctor's supervision.
>
> • Work with your doctor to determine which medication is right for you and what dosage is best.
>
> • Be aware that some medications are effective only if they are taken regularly and that symptoms may recur if the medication is stopped.
>
> Source: National Institute of Mental Health, 2009.

respond to them. Since the response is usually far less harsh than the person fears, these anxieties are lessened. People with PTSD may be supported through recalling their traumatic event in a safe situation, which helps reduce the fear it produces. CBT therapists also teach deep breathing and other types of exercises to relieve anxiety and encourage relaxation.

Exposure-based behavioral therapy has been used for many years to treat specific phobias. The person gradually encounters the object or situation that is feared, perhaps at first only through pictures or tapes, then later face-to-face. Often the therapist will accompany the person to a feared situation to provide support and guidance.

CBT is undertaken when people decide they are ready for it and with their permission and cooperation. To be effective, the therapy must be directed at the person's specific anxieties and must be tailored to his or her needs. There are no side effects other than the discomfort of temporarily increased anxiety.

CBT or behavioral therapy often lasts about 12 weeks. It may be conducted individually or with a group of people who have similar problems. Group therapy is particularly effective for social phobia. Often "homework" is assigned for participants to complete between sessions. There is some evidence that the benefits of CBT last longer than those of medication for people with panic disorder, and the same may be true for OCD, PTSD, and social phobia. If a disorder recurs at a later date, the same therapy can be used to treat it successfully a second time.

Medication can be combined with psychotherapy for specific anxiety disorders, and this is the best treatment approach for many people.

How To Get Help For Anxiety Disorders

If you think you have an anxiety disorder, the first person you should see is your family doctor. A physician can determine whether the symptoms that alarm you are due to an anxiety disorder, another medical condition, or both.

If an anxiety disorder is diagnosed, the next step is usually seeing a mental health professional. The practitioners who are most helpful with anxiety disorders are those who have training in cognitive-behavioral therapy and/or behavioral therapy, and who are open to using medication if it is needed.

You should feel comfortable talking with the mental health professional you choose. If you do not, you should seek help elsewhere. Once you find a mental health professional with whom you are comfortable, the two of you should work as a team and make a plan to treat your anxiety disorder together.

Remember that once you start on medication, it is important not to stop taking it abruptly. Certain drugs must be tapered off under the supervision of a doctor or bad reactions can occur. Make sure you talk to the doctor who prescribed your medication before you stop taking it. If you are having trouble

✎ What's It Mean?

The following types of therapy are discussed as they relate to post-traumatic stress disorder, but many also play a role in the treatment of other types of anxiety disorder.

What is group therapy?

Many people want to talk about their trauma with others who have had similar experiences.

In group therapy, you talk with a group of people who also have been through a trauma and who have post-traumatic stress disorder (PTSD). Sharing your story with others may help you feel more comfortable talking about your trauma. This can help you cope with your symptoms, memories, and other parts of your life.

Group therapy helps you build relationships with others who understand what you've been through. You learn to deal with emotions such as shame, guilt, anger, rage, and fear. Sharing with the group also can help you build self-confidence and trust. You'll learn to focus on your present life, rather than feeling overwhelmed by the past.

What is cognitive therapy?

In cognitive therapy, your therapist helps you understand and change how you think about your trauma and its aftermath. Your goal is to understand how certain thoughts about your trauma cause you stress and make your symptoms worse.

You will learn to identify thoughts about the world and yourself that are making you feel afraid or upset. With the help of your therapist, you will learn to replace these thoughts with more accurate and less distressing thoughts. You also learn ways to cope with feelings such as anger, guilt, and fear.

with side effects, it's possible that they can be eliminated by adjusting how much medication you take and when you take it.

Most insurance plans, including health maintenance organizations (HMOs), will cover treatment for anxiety disorders. Check with your insurance company and find out. If you don't have insurance, the Health and Human Services division of your county government may offer mental health care at a public mental health center that charges people according to how much they are able to pay. If you are on public assistance, you may be able to get care through your state Medicaid plan.

After a traumatic event, you might blame yourself for things you couldn't have changed. For example, a soldier may feel guilty about decisions he or she had to make during war. Cognitive therapy, a type of CBT, helps you understand that the traumatic event you lived through was not your fault.

What is exposure therapy?

In exposure therapy your goal is to have less fear about your memories. It is based on the idea that people learn to fear thoughts, feelings, and situations that remind them of a past traumatic event.

By talking about your trauma repeatedly with a therapist, you'll learn to get control of your thoughts and feelings about the trauma. You'll learn that you do not have to be afraid of your memories. This may be hard at first. It might seem strange to think about stressful things on purpose. But you'll feel less overwhelmed over time.

With the help of your therapist, you can change how you react to the stressful memories. Talking in a place where you feel secure makes this easier.

You may focus on memories that are less upsetting before talking about worse ones. This is called "desensitization," and it allows you to deal with bad memories a little bit at a time. Your therapist also may ask you to remember a lot of bad memories at once. This is called "flooding," and it helps you learn not to feel overwhelmed.

You also may practice different ways to relax when you're having a stressful memory. Breathing exercises are sometimes used for this.

Source: From "Treatment of PTSD," U.S. Department of Veterans Affairs, (www.ptsd .va.gov), November 2009.

Ways To Make Treatment More Effective

Many people with anxiety disorders benefit from joining a self-help or support group and sharing their problems and achievements with others. Internet chat rooms can also be useful in this regard, but any advice received over the internet should be used with caution, as internet acquaintances have usually never seen each other and false identities are common. Talking with a trusted friend or member of the clergy can also provide support, but it is not a substitute for care from a mental health professional.

Stress management techniques and meditation can help people with anxiety disorders calm themselves and may enhance the effects of therapy. There

---

✎ What's It Mean?

The following types of therapy are discussed as they relate to post-traumatic stress disorder, but many also play a role in the treatment of other types of anxiety disorder.

What is EMDR?

Eye movement desensitization and reprocessing (EMDR) is a fairly new therapy for post-traumatic stress disorder (PTSD). Like other kinds of counseling, it can help change how you react to memories of your trauma.

While talking about your memories, you'll focus on distractions like eye movements, hand taps, and sounds. For example, your therapist will move his or her hand near your face, and you'll follow this movement with your eyes.

Experts are still learning how EMDR works. Studies have shown that it may help you have fewer PTSD symptoms. But research also suggests that the eye movements are not a necessary part of the treatment.

What is brief psychodynamic psychotherapy?

In this type of therapy, you learn ways of dealing with emotional conflicts caused by your trauma. This therapy helps you understand how your past affects the way you feel now.

Your therapist can help you:

• Identify what triggers your stressful memories and other symptoms.

is preliminary evidence that aerobic exercise may have a calming effect. Since caffeine, certain illicit drugs, and even some over-the-counter cold medications can aggravate the symptoms of anxiety disorders, they should be avoided. Check with your physician or pharmacist before taking any additional medications.

The family is very important in the recovery of a person with an anxiety disorder. Ideally, the family should be supportive but not help perpetuate their loved one's symptoms. Family members should not trivialize the disorder or demand improvement without treatment. If your family is doing either of these things, you may want to show them this booklet so they can become educated allies and help you succeed in therapy.

- Find ways to cope with intense feelings about the past.
- Become more aware of your thoughts and feelings, so you can change your reactions to them.
- Raise your self-esteem.
- Family therapy
- Post traumatic stress disorder (PTSD) can impact your whole family. Other family members may not understand why you get angry sometimes, or why you're under so much stress. They may feel scared, guilty, or even angry about your condition.

Family therapy is a type of counseling that involves your whole family. A therapist helps you and your family communicate, maintain good relationships, and cope with tough emotions. Your family can learn more about PTSD and how it is treated.

- In family therapy, each person can express his or her fears and concerns. It's important to be honest about your feelings and to listen to others. You can talk about your PTSD symptoms and what triggers them. You also can discuss the important parts of your treatment and recovery. By doing this, your family will be better prepared to help you.

- You may consider having individual therapy for your PTSD symptoms and family therapy to help you with your relationships.

Source: From "Treatment of PTSD," U.S. Department of Veterans Affairs, (www.ptsd .va.gov), November 2009.

Role Of Research In Improving The Understanding And Treatment Of Anxiety Disorders

NIMH supports research into the causes, diagnosis, prevention, and treatment of anxiety disorders and other mental illnesses. Scientists are looking at what role genes play in the development of these disorders and are also investigating the effects of environmental factors such as pollution, physical and psychological stress, and diet. In addition, studies are being conducted on the "natural history" (what course the illness takes without treatment) of a variety of individual anxiety disorders, combinations of anxiety disorders, and anxiety disorders that are accompanied by other mental illnesses such as depression.

Scientists currently think that, like heart disease and type 1 diabetes, mental illnesses are complex and probably result from a combination of genetic, environmental, psychological, and developmental factors. For instance, although NIMH-sponsored studies of twins and families suggest that genetics play a role in the development of some anxiety disorders, problems such as PTSD are triggered by trauma. Genetic studies may help explain why some people exposed to trauma develop PTSD and others do not.

Several parts of the brain are key actors in the production of fear and anxiety. Using brain imaging technology and neurochemical techniques, scientists have discovered that the amygdala and the hippocampus play significant roles in most anxiety disorders.

The amygdala is an almond-shaped structure deep in the brain that is believed to be a communications hub between the parts of the brain that process incoming sensory signals and the parts that interpret these signals. It can alert the rest of the brain that a threat is present and trigger a fear or anxiety response. It appears that emotional memories are stored in the central part of the amygdala and may play a role in anxiety disorders involving very distinct fears, such as fears of dogs, spiders, or flying.

The hippocampus is the part of the brain that encodes threatening events into memories. Studies have shown that the hippocampus appears to be smaller in some people who were victims of child abuse or who served in military combat. Research will determine what causes this reduction in size and what role it plays in the flashbacks, deficits in explicit memory, and fragmented memories of the traumatic event that are common in PTSD.

By learning more about how the brain creates fear and anxiety, scientists may be able to devise better treatments for anxiety disorders. For example, if specific neurotransmitters are found to play an important role in fear, drugs may be developed that will block them and decrease fear responses; if enough is learned about how the brain generates new cells throughout the lifecycle, it may be possible to stimulate the growth of new neurons in the hippocampus in people with PTSD.

Chapter 13

Schizophrenia And Suicide

Schizophrenia

Schizophrenia is the most persistent and disabling of the major mental illnesses. It usually attacks people between the ages of 16 and 30, as they are beginning to realize their potential. It affects approximately one in 100 people worldwide (one per cent of the population), affecting men and women almost equally. While it is treatable in many cases, there is as yet no cure for schizophrenia.

The mind controls the basic functions of thinking, feeling (emotions), perception (the five senses), and behavior. These functions ordinarily work together, enabling us to:

- tell the difference between fantasy and reality;

- keep anxiety at manageable levels;

- have appropriate emotional responses;

- make sense of what happens to us;

- maintain a stable sense of who we are;

- establish and maintain relationships with others.

About This Chapter: This chapter includes text excerpted from "Schizophrenia," © World Fellowship for Schizophrenia and Allied Disorders, and "Warning Signs of Illness, Managing a Crisis, Risk of Suicide," © 2008 World Fellowship for Schizophrenia and Allied Disorders, http://www.worldschizophrenia.org. Reprinted with permission.

In schizophrenia, the interaction of these mental functions is disturbed in various ways.

Causes Of Schizophrenia

We do not yet understand what causes schizophrenia. Scientists generally agree that schizophrenia is a group of conditions rather than one simple disease and may therefore be found to have several causes. It is generally accepted by researchers that differences in the brain—chemical or structural, or both—may play a part in the disorder. Genetic research also suggests that while no one gene has been found for schizophrenia, several genes may cause a predisposition that can be triggered by certain life events.

> ✎ **What's It Mean?**
>
> Schizophrenia: The word schizophrenia does not mean "split personality" but a disruption of the balance among mental functions.
>
> Source: © World Fellowship for Schizophrenia and Allied Disorders.

Symptoms Of Schizophrenia

Symptoms vary greatly. Common symptoms of schizophrenia are:

Delusions: False, but strongly held beliefs, which feel entirely real to the sufferer. They can cause the individual to have a greatly exaggerated belief in his or her own importance, power, knowledge, abilities, or identity. Some people have delusions of persecution (paranoia)—for example, the false belief that they are being attacked, harassed, cheated, spied on or conspired against by others. Other people with schizophrenia believe that occurrences in the outside world are referring to them (ideas of reference). Examples are believing that other people are doing things because of you or that the TV or radio are referring specifically to you, often in negative ways.

Hallucinations: Seeing, hearing, feeling, touching smelling or tasting things that aren't there. Hallucinations have to do with the senses. Hearing voices is the most common hallucination among people with schizophrenia.

Illusions: Disturbances in perception that are less intense than hallucinations. An individual with schizophrenia may experience periods of heightened sensory awareness, during which sounds seem louder or sharper than usual and colors appear brighter, or periods of muted awareness, when sensory input seems closed off. Other illusions may include objects seeming closer or farther away than they really are, or one's own voice or reflection seeming different or even threatening.

❖ It's A Fact!!
Suicide—Always The Risk

One in ten persons suffering from schizophrenia commits suicide. Four in ten are known to have attempted suicide. Seventy percent of people who commit suicide suffer from depression. We are not telling our members anything new when we say that suicide is a serious problem; a problem that many family members have had to deal with and a problem that many families fear mightily. Yet, when we read statistics and listen to radio programs about who is most at risk we rarely hear about the large proportion of people with mental illnesses.

One statistic that we did not expect is that only 2% of those with schizophrenia who commit suicide do so in response to command voices. Young men and those with chronic illness are more at risk. A good educational background and high performance expectations are also risk factors. Some people are more aware of their illness than others and fear for the future and possible deterioration. Suicide is more likely to happen in an upswing of illness, when the symptoms have abated a little and the person sees reality more clearly. Feelings of hopelessness may run high at this time.

People often keep their thoughts of suicide very private. Rarely do professionals know how they feel. People are more likely to confide in family members, most naturally their mothers or close siblings, but some people confide in no one.

Talking about suicide should be taken seriously as it is often a plea for help. Most people who commit suicide have a history of depression or depressive features. They have taken a bleak view of the future.

Source: Excerpted from "Warning Signs of Illness, Managing a Crisis, Risk of Suicide," © 2008 World Fellowship for Schizophrenia and Allied Disorders (www.world-schizophrenia.org); reprinted with permission.

❖ **It's A Fact!!**

Risk Factors

In the general population indicators for suicide are:

• death of a loved-one;

• loss of employment;

• loss of a girlfriend/boyfriend;

• inability to work;

• feelings of worthlessness;

• divorce of family member or self may be too much to bear;

• "Copycat" effect. Hearing about a suicide may prompt the action in the person.

Family organizations have warned media not to publicize suicides to avoid this phenomenon.

Suicide may be precipitated by easy access to a means of killing oneself:

• Living high up in an apartment building

• Access to a weapon

• People often jump from bridges, throw themselves under a train or drown themselves; in rural areas, drinking pesticides is a common means.

• An overdose of medications saved up by the patient is often a method to be aware of.

When a loved-one is in hospital, be sure that staff issue day, evening, or weekend passes judiciously especially to young patients with chronic relapsing illness.

Immediately following discharge from hospital people are very vulnerable. Quite often they are not yet stable. The incidence of suicide is high among people with mental illness at this time. Careful discharge plans should be made by the hospital team and the family. If the family is not sure when the patient is to be sent home, a family member should seek this information soon after admission. Sometimes families are not advised that the patient is to be discharged.

Thought Disturbances: Often called muddled thinking by those who experience them, thought disturbances are characterized by an inability to concentrate, to connect thoughts logically, or to think clearly. Thought processes may speed up (racing thoughts) or slow down, or may seem blocked

Feelings of being alone, not having family or other support may influence a person who is already troubled. Suicide is more likely to happen when the family is away from home and leaves the ill person behind. If the person lives in the family home, try not to leave him/her alone at home for long periods if s/he seems more withdrawn or disturbed than usual. Persons living alone with few friends and very few visitors have a high incidence of suicide. If this is your situation, visit, phone or mail postcards or greetings cards regularly to keep in contact. Access to the Internet can be a source of social contact for people living alone. Be particularly suspicious when someone's previously gloomy mood suddenly changes to cheerfulness without sufficient reason. This may apply, but might be difficult to define in someone with bipolar disorder.

People sometimes write poems, notes or other material dwelling on death or suicide when they are contemplating these. An informal study of local suicides prompted one group to suggest being especially vigilant and considerate of your relative in the Spring or at family festival times. This may be because Spring is a symbol of renewal and at family festival times one experiences first hand the achievements of other family members. The person's own feelings of unhappiness may become overwhelming.

If the person lives at home, set up realistic rules for home life to help the family live as "smoothly" as possible. This may be helpful for your relative who is dealing with incredibly difficult symptoms.

Issues of suicide should be addressed directly. Acknowledge with empathy the patient's view that death is one solution to the problem of the unbearable psychological pain. Give your relative hope by speaking of the many advances in research and the better medications that will soon be available. Tell him/her that you want him/her to be around to benefit from these.

Source: Excerpted from "Warning Signs of Illness, Managing a Crisis, Risk of Suicide," © 2008 World Fellowship for Schizophrenia and Allied Disorders (www .world-schizophrenia.org); reprinted with permission.

so that the person's mind feels completely blank. Disturbances in thinking are sometimes compared to a broken filter that allows everything that enters the mind to have the same importance—for example, attaching the same significance to license plate numbers as to a questions from a teacher.

Emotional And Behavioral Changes: A person with schizophrenia can experience sudden, inexplicable changes in mood, such as intense sadness, happiness, excitement, depression, or anger that come on without reason or warning. Lack of feelings can be equally disturbing. Symptoms that deprive a person of a range of normal emotions are often described as "negative." The person seems less able to feel anything, including pain or joy. Sometimes this loss of feeling extends to the "sense of self." The individual experiences a sense of unreality about who and where they are or where their body ends. More than any of the symptoms described above, the behavioral changes indicate to others the possible presence of schizophrenia.

An early sign of disturbance is often social withdrawal, as the individual finds interactions with people and things progressively more difficult. One such common response is inability to take an interest in personal hygiene and appearance. Lack of energy, interest and motivation or decreased levels of activity, movement or speech should alert friends and family that something may be amiss. Similarly, behavior patterns that are unusual in the particular individual, or responses that are clearly inappropriate (excessive laughing or crying in inappropriate circumstances, or excessive talking to oneself) may indicate the approach of an episode of schizophrenia.

Treating Schizophrenia

New medications for schizophrenia along with better prescribing practices (more appropriate dosing), make treatment more successful than in the past. Schizophrenia is treated with medications called antipsychotics. In the last 10 years new compounds have been introduced that have a significantly reduced side-effect profile. In addition it has been recognized that stabilization and recovery from schizophrenia are significantly enhanced with the complimentary treatment of social, employment, and family supports.

Antipsychotic medications work on several levels. They can have an immediate calming effect, reducing anxiety, agitation and restlessness in the person with symptoms of schizophrenia. It can take up to four weeks to reduce symptoms such as hallucinations. Thought disturbances and paranoia are more resistant to medications.

Some people are unwilling to take tablets, even for a short period, because they do not believe they are ill, or because of a previous unpleasant experience with medication. In addition to tablets, medications are also available by injection every two to three weeks. These are especially helpful for people who forget to take their pills.

People with schizophrenia are particularly vulnerable and need social supports—decent housing, income support, supportive friends and family, and something worthwhile to do. Most people with schizophrenia become ill at the age they would be making career choices, undergoing training and forming adult relationships. As a result, they often lack social and work skills. So in addition to medication, people with schizophrenia may need training in social skills, money management and problem solving. Those who can work often need further training and employment support.

Risk Of Suicide

Families must always be aware that there can be a high risk for suicide in people with schizophrenia. One in 10 people with schizophrenia commit suicide and four in 10 attempt to end their lives.

Chapter 14

Abuse Of Alcohol And Other Substances Increases Suicide Risk

Substance Use Disorders And Suicide

A growing body of studies has demonstrated that alcohol and drug abuse are second only to depression and other mood disorders as the most frequent risk factors for suicide. Data from the National Comorbidity Survey disclosed that alcohol and drug abuse disorders are associated with a risk 6.2 times greater than average risk of suicide attempts.

According to the Substance Abuse and Mental Health Services Administration (SAMHSA)'s Drug Abuse Warning Network latest report on drug-related emergency department (ED) visits, in 2005, over 132,500 visits to emergency rooms were for alcohol- or drug-related suicide attempts. Substantial percentages of suicide victims tested positive for alcohol or other drugs. The most frequently identified substance was alcohol, found in one third of those tested; four other substances were identified in approximately

About This Chapter: This chapter begins with excerpts from *Substance Abuse and Suicide Prevention: Evidence and Implications—A White Paper*, Center for Substance Abuse Treatment, DHHS Pub. No. SMA-08-4352. Rockville, MD: Substance Abuse and Mental Health Services Administration, 2008. It continues with information from "Depression Elevates Suicide Risk in Substance-Abusing Adolescents," *NIDA Notes*, National Institute on Drug Abuse, Vol. 19, No. 6 (May 2005); and "Twin Study Links Marijuana Abuse, Suicide, And Depression Research Findings," by Patrick Zickler, *NIDA Notes*, Vol. 20, No. 2 (August 2005).

10 percent of tested victims. Illicit drugs were involved in approximately one fifth (19%) of the ED visits for drug-related suicide attempts. Over 85 percent of individuals associated with these attempts were seriously ill enough to merit admission to a hospital or anot.her health care facility.

The Drug Abuse Warning Network also has examined emergency department visits for drug-related suicide attempts by youth. In 2004, the most recent year for which data are available, reporting emergency departments handled over 15,000 drug-related suicide attempts by youth, ages 12–17, almost 75 percent of which were serious enough to warrant hospitalization.

These data do not suggest that all of the individuals who attempted suicide, whether young or adult, were experiencing substance abuse disorders; rather the data inform only that alcohol or drugs of abuse were used in what was characterized as a suicide attempt. Nonetheless, the sheer numbers are compelling.

Field-based studies have been ongoing to understand the relationships between substances of abuse and suicide. Significant studies have been based on psychological autopsies; only in the last few years have increasing numbers of prospective studies been conducted. Research is complicated and sometimes confounded by the complex interrelationships among mental and substance use disorders, combined with other biological, behavioral, environmental and social factors influencing suicide risk.

Alcohol: As many as one fourth of individuals who die by suicide are intoxicated with alcohol. The association between suicidal behavior and alcohol abuse has been long documented, dating back to the 1980s. An extensive body of literature has established that active alcohol use or abuse is a powerful risk factor for suicide. One of the more significant reasons posited for this association is the disinhibition resulting from alcohol use that occurs shortly prior to a suicide attempt. Another study suggests that the role of alcohol in suicidal behavior may include promoting depression and hopelessness, impairing problem solving, and facilitating aggression.

Drugs: Relatively little is known about the impact of different drugs, drug combinations, substance-induced effects, and self-medication on suicidal behavior. What is known is that there is some association between current drug

✤ It's A Fact!!
Alcohol And Suicide Among Racial/Ethnic Populations

From 2001 to 2005, there were an estimated annual 79,646 alcohol attributable deaths and 2.3 million years of potential life was lost attributed to the harmful effects of excessive alcohol use. The burden of suicide varies widely among racial and ethnic populations in the United States, and limited data is available to describe the role of alcohol in suicides in these populations. To examine the relationship between alcohol and suicide among racial/ethnic populations, Centers for Disease Control and Prevention analyzed data from the National Violent Death Reporting System (NVDRS) for a two-year period between 2005 and 2006. The results indicate that many populations can benefit from comprehensive and culturally appropriate suicide-prevention strategies that include efforts to reduce alcohol consumption, especially programs that focus on individuals under 50 years old.

Effective, comprehensive suicide-prevention programs have been developed. These programs focus on an array of risk or protective factors, including alcohol consumption, substance misuse, and social support; however, few have been developed specifically for minority populations. Some international studies suggest that measures to restrict alcohol use can reduce suicides. The measures include raising the minimum legal drinking age, increasing taxes on alcohol sales, limiting the sale of alcohol products by age of purchaser, time of day available, or business type, and mandating that workplaces be alcohol-free. Other program components include outreach to families after a suicide or traumatic death, immediate response and follow-up for reported at-risk youth, alcohol and substance abuse programs, community education about suicide prevention, and suicide-risk screening in mental health and social service programs.

Source: Excerpted from "Alcohol and Suicide Among Racial/Ethnic Populations—17 States, 2005–2006," reported by AE Crosby, MD; V Espitia-Hardeman, MSc; HA Hill, MD, PhD; L Ortega, MD; and C Clavel-Arcas, MD; National Center for Injury Prevention and Control, CDC. *MMWR*, June 19, 2009/58(23);637–641.

use and suicidal ideation that is not entirely due to the effects of co-occurring mental disorders. The number of substances used appears to be more predictive of suicidal behavior than the types of substances used. Moreover, based on a few initial studies, it also appears that drug abuse treatment itself may have the capacity to help reduce the risk for future suicidality.

Co-Occurring Disorders: A substantial body of knowledge suggests that substance use—both drugs and alcohol—is associated with mental disorders. Moreover, some suggest that this linkage may be bidirectional. For example, depression may be associated with increased substance use and chronic substance abuse may be a factor in the development of depression or other mood disorders.

Further, both mental and substance use disorders are known risk factors for suicide. Secondary analysis of combined 2004 and 2005 data from SAMHSA's National Survey on Drug Use and Health (NSDUH) sheds light not only on the magnitude of co-occurring mental and substance use disorders, but also on the considerable impact they have when they occur together. According to the NSDUH analysis, an estimated 16.4 million adults, age 18 and older, experienced a major depressive episode in the past year. During their worst or most recent experience of major depression, over half thought they would be better off dead; over 10 percent attempted suicide. When alcohol abuse or the use of illicit drugs was added to a major depressive episode, the proportion of suicide attempts rose to nearly 14 percent for alcohol abuse and nearly 20 percent for illicit drug use.

Depression Elevates Suicide Risk In Substance-Abusing Adolescents

A recent study funded by the National Institute on Drug Abuse (NIDA) highlights the need for substance abuse counselors to be aware of depression and suicide risk in their adolescent patients. Drs. Thomas Kelly, Duncan Clark, and colleagues at the University of Pittsburgh School of Medicine identified 85 suicide attempters in a series of 503 substance-abusing teenagers studied from 1991 to 2000. Most of the teenagers abused alcohol (88 percent) and marijuana (80 percent). A large majority—87 percent—of those who had attempted suicide were diagnosed with major depression using the *Diagnostic and Statistical Manual, 4th Edition* (*DSM-IV*) criteria. Among substance-abusing teens who did not attempt suicide, major depression was diagnosed in only 40 percent. Girls were three times more likely to have attempted suicide than boys. Among the attempters, one-third of girls and one-tenth of boys reported multiple attempts—a finding consistent with general patterns of suicidal behaviors.

♣ It's A Fact!!

"The connection between substance abuse and suicide has not been sufficiently well understood," said Richard McKeon, Ph.D., M.P.H., Public Health Adviser for Suicide Prevention at the Substance Abuse and Mental Health Services Administration (SAMHSA)'s Center for Mental Health Services. "People in both the mental health and substance abuse fields have likely had experiences that would demonstrate the connection, but I think that probably few appreciate the magnitude of the relationship between substance abuse and suicide."

Because of cultural taboos it has only been in the last decade or so that the public health field has focused its attention on suicide. With the realization that people with mental health and substance abuse disorders can recover has come the recognition that people at risk for suicide can be treated.

What's needed is an approach that targets the entire population, relies on best practices, and addresses the full range of risk factors, adding substance abuse to better-known risk factors such as mental illness and certain biological and environmental characteristics. The approach should focus on prevention just as much as diagnosis and treatment.

"There's a need for a comprehensive approach if we want to reduce suicide attempts and death by suicide," emphasized Dr. McKeon. "It's not sufficient to rely simply on mental health treatment, since we know that the majority of those who die by suicide have never had any mental health treatment. To reduce suicide, everyone needs to be involved."

Source: Excerpted from "Substance Abuse and Suicide: White Paper Explores Connection," by Rebecca A. Clay, *SAMHSA News*, Vol. 17, No. 1, January/February 2009.

"Clinicians who work with adolescent substance abusers may not automatically think about suicidal behavior as something to watch for in their clients, but it's definitely a concern—especially for youth with co-occurring psychiatric disorders," says Dr. Lynda Erinoff of NIDA's Division of Epidemiology, Services and Prevention Research. There is an association between substance abuse, co-occurring psychiatric disorders, and suicidal behavior in adults and adolescents, but Dr. Erinoff explains that it's difficult to establish causal factors and sequencing of these problems.

Twin Study Links Marijuana Abuse, Suicide, And Depression

Men and women who smoked marijuana before age 17 are 3.5 times as likely to attempt suicide as those who started later. Individuals who are dependent on marijuana have a higher risk than nondependent individuals of experiencing major depressive disorder and suicidal thoughts and behaviors. The researchers who discovered these relationships, in a recent NIDA-funded large-scale epidemiological study, say that although the causes are not clear, their findings demonstrate the importance of considering associated mental health issues in the treatment and prevention of marijuana abuse.

Dr. Michael Lynskey and colleagues at the Washington University School of Medicine in St. Louis, Missouri, gathered data from four groups of same-sex twin pairs (508 identical, 493 fraternal; 518 female, 483 male) enrolled in the Australian Twin Registry:

• Among the 277 pairs who were discordant for marijuana dependence (that is, one twin but not the other met the criteria for a diagnosis of marijuana dependence), the dependent twins were 2.9 times as likely as their nondependent co-twins to think about suicide without attempting it, and 2.5 times as likely to make a suicide attempt.

• Among the 311 pairs discordant for early marijuana initiation (just one twin in each pair smoked marijuana before age 17), the early initiators were 3.5 times as likely as their twins to attempt suicide, but no more likely to suffer a major depressive disorder (MDD).

• Among the 156 pairs discordant for diagnosis of major depressive disorder (MDD) before age 17, fraternal but not identical twins with early diagnosis of MDD were 9.5 times as likely to develop marijuana dependence.

• Among the 257 pairs discordant for having suicidal thoughts before age 17, fraternal but not identical twins with early suicidal thoughts were 5.5 times as likely as their twins to become dependent on marijuana.

"Overall, the associations between marijuana abuse and depressive disorders suggest a relationship that is contributory but not necessarily causal. Depressive disorders in and of themselves do not cause people to abuse marijuana, and marijuana abuse and dependence do not of themselves cause depression or suicidal behavior," Dr. Lynskey says. "Nevertheless, clinicians treating patients for one disorder should take the other into account at initial assessment and throughout treatment. In the context of treatment, both need to be addressed, because it is not necessarily the case that eliminating one disorder will get rid of the other." The fact that two of the relationships were observed in fraternal but not identical twins suggests that the experiences related in each—marijuana dependence and MDD, and marijuana dependence and suicidal thoughts—may share a common underlying genetic basis, notes Dr. Lynskey.

The associations identified in this study are complex, but point to a simple policy implication, observes Dr. Lynskey. "It is important to see that prevention efforts aimed at one disorder may well have the additional benefit of preventing or reducing the other," he says.

"Drug abuse and depression co-occur at rates much greater than chance and constitute a serious public health concern," says Dr. Naimah Weinberg of NIDA's Division of Epidemiology, Services and Prevention Research. "Understanding how each disorder may contribute to the development and course of the other, and what factors may underlie their co-occurrence, has important implications for prevention and treatment of these disabling conditions."

Chapter 15

Abusing Prescription And Over-The-Counter Drugs

Prescription Drug Abuse

Angie overheard her parents talking about how her brother's attention deficit hyperactivity disorder (ADHD) medicine was making him less hungry. Because Angie was worried about her weight, she started sneaking one of her brother's pills every few days. To prevent her parents from finding out, she asked a friend to give her some of his ADHD medicine as well.

Todd found an old bottle of painkillers that had been left over from his dad's operation. He decided to try them. Because a doctor had prescribed the pills, Todd figured that meant they'd be OK to try.

Both Todd and Angie are taking huge risks, though. Prescription painkillers and other medications help lots of people live more productive lives, freeing them from the symptoms of medical conditions like depression or attention deficit hyperactivity disorder. But that's only when they're prescribed for a particular individual to treat a specific condition.

About This Chapter: "Prescription Drug Abuse," November 2009, reprinted with permission from www.kidshealth.org. Copyright © 2009 The Nemours Foundation. This information was provided by KidsHealth, one of the largest resources online for medically reviewed health information written for parents, kids, and teens. For more articles like this one, visit www.KidsHealth.org, or www.TeensHealth.org.

Taking prescription drugs in a way that hasn't been recommended by a doctor can be more dangerous than people think. In fact, it's drug abuse. And it's just as illegal as taking street drugs.

Why Do Some People Abuse Prescription Drugs?

Some people experiment with prescription drugs because they think they will help them have more fun, lose weight, fit in, and even study more effectively. Prescription drugs can be easier to get than street drugs: Family members or friends could have a prescription. But prescription drugs are also sometimes sold on the street like other illegal drugs. A 2006 National Survey on Drug Use and Health showed that among all youths aged 12 to 17, 6% had tried prescription drugs for recreational use in the last month.

> ❖ **It's A Fact!!**
> **Drug Poisoning**
>
> Overdosing isn't the only way drugs can kill. We know from basic science that chemical and compounds sometimes react with each other. So it can be risky, even deadly, to take certain directions on each medication. And avoid taking someone else's prescription, even if you have the same condition.

Why? Some people think that prescription drugs are safer and less addictive than street drugs. After all, these are drugs that moms, dads, and even kid brothers and sisters use. To Angie, taking her brother's ADHD medicine felt like a good way to keep her appetite in check. She'd heard how bad diet pills can be, and she wrongly thought that the ADHD drugs would be safer.

But prescription drugs are only safe for the individuals who actually have prescriptions for them. That's because a doctor has examined these people and prescribed the right dose of medication for a specific medical condition. The doctor has also told them exactly how they should take the medicine, including things to avoid while taking the drug—such as drinking alcohol, smoking, or taking other medications. They also are aware of potentially dangerous side effects and can monitor patients closely for these.

Other people who try prescription drugs are like Todd. They think they're not doing anything illegal because these drugs are prescribed by doctors. But taking drugs without a prescription — or sharing a prescription drug with friends—is actually breaking the law.

Which Drugs Are Abused?

The most commonly used prescription drugs fall into three classes:

1. Opioids

- **Examples:** Oxycodone (OxyContin), hydrocodone (Vicodin), and meperidine (Demerol)
- **Medical Uses:** Opioids are used to treat pain or relieve coughs or diarrhea.
- **How They Work:** Opioids attach to opioid receptors in the central nervous system (the brain and the spinal cord), preventing the brain from receiving pain messages.

2. Central Nervous System (CNS) Depressants

- **Examples:** Pentobarbital sodium (Nembutal), diazepam (Valium), and alprazolam (Xanax)
- **Medical Uses:** CNS depressants are used to treat anxiety, tension, panic attacks, and sleep disorders.
- **How They Work:** CNS depressants slow down brain activity by increasing the activity of a neurotransmitter called GABA. The result is a drowsy or calming effect.

3. Stimulants

- **Examples:** Methylphenidate (Ritalin) and amphetamine/dextroamphetamine (Adderall)
- **Medical Uses:** Stimulants can be used to treat narcolepsy and ADHD.
- **How They Work:** Stimulants increase brain activity, resulting in greater alertness, attention, and energy.

Over-The-Counter Drugs

Some people mistakenly think that prescription drugs are more powerful because you need a prescription for them. But it's possible to abuse or become addicted to over-the-counter (OTC) medications, too.

For example, dextromethorphan (DXM) is found in some OTC cough medicines. When someone takes the number of teaspoons or tablets that are recommended, everything is fine. But high doses can cause problems with the senses (especially vision and hearing) and can lead to confusion, stomach pain, numbness, and even hallucinations.

> ✦ **It's A Fact!!**
> **Where's The**
> **Cold Medicine?**
>
> In some parts of the country, you can only get over the counter cold medications in limited quantities from a pharmacist. That's because some of the ingredients they contain can be used by illegal drug labs to make dangerous street drugs like methamphetamine.

What Are The Dangers Of Abusing Medications?

Whether they're using street drugs or medications, drug abusers often have trouble at school, at home, with friends, or with the law. The likelihood that someone will commit a crime, be a victim of a crime, or have an accident is higher when that person is abusing drugs—no matter whether those drugs are medications or street drugs.

Like all drug abuse, using prescription drugs for the wrong reasons has serious risks for a person's health. Opioid abuse can lead to vomiting, mood changes, decrease in ability to think (cognitive function), and even decreased respiratory function, coma, or death. This risk is higher when prescription drugs like opioids are taken with other substances like alcohol, antihistamines, and CNS depressants.

CNS depressants have risks, too. Abruptly stopping or reducing them too quickly can lead to seizures. Taking CNS depressants with other medications, such as prescription painkillers, some over-the-counter cold and allergy medications, or alcohol can slow a person's heartbeat and breathing—and even kill.

Abusing stimulants (like some ADHD drugs) may cause heart failure or seizures. These risks are increased when stimulants are mixed with other medicines—even OTC ones like certain cold medicines. Taking too much of a stimulant can lead a person to develop a dangerously high body temperature or an irregular heartbeat. Taking several high doses over a short period of time may make a drug abuser aggressive or paranoid.

Although stimulant abuse might not lead to physical dependence and withdrawal, the feelings these drugs give people can cause them to use the drugs more and more often so they become a habit that's hard to break.

The dangers of prescription drug abuse can be made even worse if people take drugs in a way they weren't intended to be used. Ritalin may seem harmless because it's prescribed even for little kids with ADHD. But when a person takes it either unnecessarily or in a way it wasn't intended to be used such as snorting or injection, Ritalin toxicity can be serious. And because there can be many variations of the same medication, the dose of medication and how long it stays in the body can vary. The person who doesn't have a prescription might not really know which one he or she has.

Probably the most common result of prescription drug abuse is addiction. People who abuse medications can become addicted just as easily as if they were taking street drugs. The reason many drugs have to be prescribed by a doctor is because some of them are quite addictive. That's one of the reasons most doctors won't usually renew a prescription unless they see the patient—they want to examine the patient to make sure he or she isn't getting addicted.

How Do I Know If I'm Addicted?

Many different signs can point to drug addiction. The most obvious is feeling the need to have a particular drug or substance. Changes in mood, weight, or interests are other signs of drug addiction.

If you think you—or a friend—may be addicted to prescription drugs, talk to your doctor, school counselor, or nurse. They can help you get the help you need. It's especially important for someone who is going through withdrawal from a CNS depressant to speak with a doctor or seek medical treatment. Withdrawal can be dangerous when it's not monitored.

If someone has become addicted to prescription drugs, there are several kinds of treatment, depending on individual needs and the type of drug used. The two main categories of drug addiction treatment are behavioral and pharmacological.

Behavioral treatments teach people how to function without drugs— handling cravings, avoiding drugs and situations that could lead to drug use, and preventing and handling relapses. Pharmacological treatments involve giving patients a special type of medication to help them overcome withdrawal symptoms and drug cravings.

Tips For Taking Prescription Medication

What if a doctor prescribed a medication for you and you're worried about becoming addicted? If you're taking the medicine the way your doctor told you to, you can relax: Doctors know how much medication to prescribe so that it's just enough for you. In the correct amount, the drug will relieve your symptoms without making you addicted.

If a doctor prescribes a pain medication, stimulant, or CNS depressant, follow the directions exactly.

Finally, never use someone else's prescription. And don't allow a friend to use yours. Not only are you putting your friend at risk, but you could suffer, too: Pharmacists won't refill a prescription if a medication has been used up before it should be. And if you're found giving medication to someone else, it's considered a crime and you could find yourself in court.

☞ Remember!!

Here are some other ways to protect yourself:

- Keep all doctor's appointments. Your doctor will want you to visit often so he or she can monitor how well the medication is working for you and adjust the dose or change the medication as needed. Some medications must be stopped or changed after a while so that the person doesn't become addicted.

- Make a note of the effects the drug has on your body and emotions, especially in the first few days as your body gets used to it. Tell your doctor about these.

- Keep any information your pharmacist gives you about any drugs or activities you should steer clear of while taking your prescription. Reread it often to remind yourself of what you should avoid. If the information is too long or complicated, ask a parent or your pharmacist to give you the highlights.

- Don't increase or decrease the dose of your medication without checking with your doctor's office first—no matter how you're feeling.

Chapter 16

Abusive Relationships May Increase Suicide Risk

Lots Of Relationships Turn Abusive

When Brian and Sarah began dating, her friends were envious. Brian was smart, sensitive, funny, athletic, and good-looking.

For the first couple of months, Sarah seemed happy. She started to miss her friends and family, though, because she was spending more time with Brian and less time with everyone else. That seemed easier than dealing with Brian's endless questions. He worried about what she was doing at every moment of the day.

Sarah's friends became concerned when her behavior started to change. She lost interest in the things she once enjoyed, like swim meets and going to the mall. She became secretive and moody. When her friends asked if she was having trouble with Brian, she denied that anything was wrong.

Healthy relationships involve respect, trust, and consideration for the other person. Sadly, lots of relationships don't have these qualities—and many turn abusive. In fact, one in 11 high school students report being physically hurt by a date.

About This Chapter: "Abusive Relationships," November 2007, reprinted with permission from www.kidshealth.org. Copyright © 2007 The Nemours Foundation. This information was provided by KidsHealth, one of the largest resources online for medically reviewed health information written for parents, kids, and teens. For more articles like this one, visit www.KidsHealth.org, or www.TeensHealth.org.

People in abusive relationships sometimes mistake the abuse for intense feelings of caring or concern. It can even seem flattering. Think of a friend whose boyfriend or girlfriend is insanely jealous: Maybe it seems like your friend's partner really cares. But actually, excessive jealousy and controlling behavior are not signs of affection at all. Love involves respect and trust; it doesn't mean constantly worrying about the possible end of the relationship.

What Is Abuse?

Abuse can be physical, emotional, or sexual. Slapping, hitting, and kicking are forms of physical abuse that can occur in both romances and friendships.

Emotional abuse (stuff like teasing, bullying, and humiliating others) can be difficult to recognize because it doesn't leave any visible scars. Threats, intimidation, putdowns, and betrayal are all harmful forms of emotional abuse that can really hurt—not just during the time it's happening, but long after too.

> ✤ **It's A Fact!!**
> **How does dating violence affect health?**
>
> Dating violence can have a negative effect on health throughout life. Teens who are victims are more likely to do poorly in school. They may engage in unhealthy behaviors, like drug and alcohol use. The anger and stress that victims feel may lead to eating disorders and depression. Some teens even think about or attempt suicide.
>
> Source: Excerpted from "Understanding Teen Dating Violence," National Center for Injury Prevention and Control, Centers for Disease Control and Prevention (www.cdc.gov/violenceprevention), 2009.

Sexual abuse can happen to anyone, guy or girl. It's never right to be forced into any type of sexual experience that you don't want.

The first step in getting out of an abusive relationship is to realize that you have the right to be treated with respect and not be physically or emotionally harmed by another person.

Signs Of Abusive Relationships

Important warning signs that you may be involved in an abusive relationship include when someone:

- harms you physically in any way, including slapping, pushing, grabbing, shaking, smacking, kicking, and punching;

- tries to control different aspects of your life, such as how you dress, who you hang out with, and what you say;

- frequently humiliates you or making you feel unworthy (for example, if a partner puts you down but tells you that he or she loves you);

- coerces or threatens to harm you, or self-harm, if you leave the relationship;

- twists the truth to make you feel you are to blame for your partner's actions;

- demands to know where you are at all times;

- constantly becomes jealous or angry when you want to spend time with your friends.

Unwanted sexual advances that make you uncomfortable are also red flags that the relationship needs to focus more on respect. When someone says stuff like "If you loved me, you would . . . " that's also a warning of possible abuse. A statement like this is controlling and is used by people who are only concerned about getting what they want—not caring about what you want. Trust your intuition. If something doesn't feel right, it probably isn't.

✤ It's A Fact!!
How does sexual violence affect health?

Sexual violence can impact health in many ways. Some ways are serious and can lead to long-term health problems. These include chronic pain, headaches, stomach problems, and sexually transmitted diseases.

Sexual violence can have emotional impact as well. Victims often are fearful and anxious. They may replay the attack over and over in their minds. They may have problems with trust and be wary of becoming involved with others. The anger and stress that victims feel may lead to eating disorders and depression. Some even think about or attempt suicide.

Sexual violence is also linked to negative health behaviors. For example, victims are more likely to smoke, abuse alcohol, use drugs, and engage in risky sexual activity.

Source: Excerpted from "Understanding Sexual Violence," National Center for Injury Prevention and Control, Centers for Disease Control and Prevention (www.cdc.gov/violenceprevention), 2009.

Signs That A Friend Is Being Abused

In addition to the signs listed above, here are some signs a friend might be being abused by a partner:

- unexplained bruises, broken bones, sprains, or marks;
- excessive guilt or shame for no apparent reason;
- secrecy or withdrawal from friends and family;
- avoidance of school or social events with excuses that don't seem to make any sense.

A person who is being abused needs someone to hear and believe him or her. Maybe your friend is afraid to tell a parent because that will bring pressure to end the relationship. People who are abused often feel like it's their fault—that they "asked for it" or that they don't deserve any better. But abuse is never deserved. Help your friend understand that it is not his or her fault. Your friend is not a bad person. The person who is being abusive has a serious problem and needs professional help.

A friend who is being abused needs your patience, love, and understanding. Your friend also needs your encouragement to get help immediately from an adult, such as a parent or guidance counselor. Most of all, your friend needs you to listen without judging. It takes a lot of courage to admit being abused; let your friend know that you're offering your full support.

How You Can Help Yourself

What should you do if you are suffering from any type of abuse? If you think you love someone but often feel afraid, it's time to get out of the relationship—fast. You're worth being treated with respect and you can get help.

First, make sure you're safe. A trusted adult can help. If the person has physically attacked you, don't wait to get medical attention or to call the police. Assault is illegal, and so is rape—even if it's done by someone you are dating.

Avoid the tendency to isolate yourself from your friends and family. You might feel like you have nowhere to turn, or you might be embarrassed about what's been going on, but this is when you need support most. People like counselors, doctors, teachers, coaches, and friends will want to help you, so let them.

Don't rely on yourself alone to get out of the situation. Friends and family who love and care about you can help you break away. It's important to know that asking for help isn't a sign of weakness. It actually shows that you have a lot of courage and are willing to stand up for yourself.

Where To Get Help

Ending abuse and violence in teen relationships is a community effort with plenty of people ready to help. Your local phone book will list crisis centers, teen help lines, and abuse hotlines. These organizations have professionally trained staff to listen, understand, and help. In addition, religious leaders, school nurses, teachers, school counselors, doctors, and other health professionals can be sources of support and information.

You can also get involved at a school or community level as an advocate to help prevent future dating abuse. One example of a school-based program is Safe Dates. Talk to your school guidance counselor about starting a group or other ways to get involved in making sure dating abuse doesn't happen to people in your school.

Abuse has no place in love.

Chapter 17

Self-Injury In Teens

The number of young people who participate in acts of self-mutilation is growing. Although self-harm is rarely a suicidal act, it must be taken seriously because accidental deaths do occur. It's difficult to see the light at the end of the tunnel, but breaking the cycle of self-abuse is possible if you reach out to someone you trust. Finding new ways of coping with your feelings can help to tone down the intense urges you feel which results in you hurting yourself. Recovery is a continuous process and learning how to stop this addictive behavior is within your reach if you work at it.

Who Engages In Self-Injury?

The numbers are staggering. About two million people in the U.S. are self-injurers and approximately 1% of the population has inflicted physical injury upon themselves at some time in their life as a way to cope with an overwhelming situation or feeling. Those numbers are most likely an underestimation because the majority of acts of self-injury go unreported. In other parts of the world the numbers are considerably higher. Self-injury

About This Chapter: Text in this chapter is from "Cutting and Self-Injury," by Deborah Cutter, Psy.D., Jaelline Jaffe, Ph.D., and Jeanne Segal, Ph.D., reprinted with permission from http://helpguide.org/mental/self_injury.htm. © 2008 Helpguide.org. All rights reserved. Helpguide provides a detailed list of related references for this article, including links to information from other websites. For a complete list of Helpguide's current resources related to self-injury, including information about suicide, stress management, and mental health, visit www.helpguide.org.

does not discriminate against race, culture, or socioeconomic strata, but there is conflicting data regarding demographics. Some reference sites indicate that the majority of people who engage in this type of addictive behavior are predominately female teenagers and young adults, while other sites indicate that both genders, ranging in age from 14 to 60 self-injure. However, there is consistent agreement that self-harm has more to do with having poor coping mechanisms than anything else.

Reasons For Self-Injury

Even though it is possible that a self-inflicted injury may result in death, self-injury is usually not suicidal behavior. The person who self-injures may not recognize the connection, but this act usually occurs after an overwhelming or distressing experience and is a result of not having learned how to identify or express difficult feelings in a healthy way. Sometimes the person who deliberately harms themselves thinks that if they feel the pain on the outside instead of feeling it on the inside, the injuries will be seen, which then perhaps gives them a fighting chance to heal. They may also believe that the wounds, which are now physical evidence, proves their emotional pain is real. Although the physical pain they experience may be the catalyst that releases the emotional pain, the relief they feel is temporary. These coping mechanisms in essence are faulty because the pain eventually returns without any permanent healing taking place.

> ♣ **It's A Fact!!**
> Self-harm serves a function for the person who does it. If you can figure out what function the self-injury is serving then you can learn other ways to get those needs met which will reduce your desire to hurt yourself.

It is difficult to understand the motivations behind self-injurious behavior, but a clearer picture develops when you hear the common explanations self-injurers give for doing it:

- "It expresses emotional pain or feelings that I'm unable to put into words. It puts a punctuation mark on what I'm feeling on the inside!"

- "It's a way to have control over my body because I can't control anything else in my life."

✎ What's It Mean?

Self-Injury: Self-injury, self-inflicted violence, self-injurious behavior, or self-mutilation is defined as a deliberate, intentional injury to one's own body that causes tissue damage or leaves marks for more than a few minutes which is done to cope with an overwhelming or distressing situation.

The most common self-injurious behaviors are:

- **Cutting:** Involves making cuts or scratches on your body with any sharp object, including knives, needles, razor blades, or even fingernails. The arms, legs, and front of the torso are most commonly cut because they are easily reached and easily hidden under clothing.

- **Branding:** Burning self with a hot object.

- **Friction Burn:** Rubbing a pencil eraser on your skin.

- **Picking At Skin** or re-opening wounds (dermatillomania): Is an impulse control disorder characterized by the repeated urge to pick at one's own skin, often to the extent that damage is caused which relieves stress or is gratifying.

- **Hair-Pulling** (trichotillomania): Is an impulse control disorder which at times seems to resemble a habit, an addiction, or an obsessive-compulsive disorder. The person has an irresistible urge to pull out hair from any part of their body. Hair pulling from the scalp often leaves patchy bald spots on their head which they hide by wearing hats, scarves, and wigs. Abnormal levels of serotonin or dopamine may play a role in this disorder. The combined treatment of using an antidepressant such as Anafranil and cognitive behavioral therapy (CBT) has been effective in treating this disorder. CBT teaches you to become more aware of when you're pulling, helps you identify your pulling habits, and teaches you about what emotions and triggers are involved in hair pulling. When you gain awareness of pulling, you can learn to substitute healthier behaviors instead.

- **Hitting** (with hammer or other object), **Bone Breaking, Punching, Head-Banging** (more often seen with autism or severe mental retardation).

- **Multiple Piercing Or Tattooing:** May also be a type of self-injury, especially if pain or stress relief is a factor.

- **Drinking Harmful Chemicals.**

- "I usually feel like I have a black hole in the pit of my stomach, at least if I feel pain it's better than feeling nothing."

- "I feel relieved and less anxious after I cut. The emotional pain slowly slips away into the physical pain."

Self-injury can regulate strong emotions. It can put a person who is at a high level of physiological arousal back to a baseline state.

Deliberate self-harm can distract from emotional pain and stop feelings of numbness.

Self-inflicted violence is a way to express things that cannot be put into words such as displaying anger, shocking others, or seeking support and help.

Self-injurious behavior can exert a sense of control over your body if you feel powerless in other areas of your life. Sometimes magical thinking is involved and you may imagine that hurting yourself will prevent something worse from happening. Also, when you hurt yourself it influences the behavior of others and can manipulate people into feeling guilty, make them care, or make them go away.

Self punishment or self-hate may be involved. Some people who self-injure have a childhood history of physical, sexual, and emotional abuse. They may errone-ously blame themselves for having been abused, they may feel that they deserved it and are now punishing themselves because of self-hatred and low self-esteem.

Self-abuse can also be a self-soothing behavior for someone who does not have other means to calm intense emotions. Self-injury followed by tending to one's own wounds is a way to express self-care and be self-nurturing for someone who never learned how to do that in a more direct way.

People who self-injure have some common traits:

- Expressions of anger were discouraged while growing up

- They have co-existing problems with obsessive-compulsive disorder, substance abuse, or eating disorders

- They lack the necessary skills to express strong emotions in a healthy way

- Often times there is a limited social support network

Self-Injury As An Addiction

Becoming a habitual self injurer is a progressive process. The first incident of self-injury may occur by accident, or after finding out about others who engage in this behavior.

- The person has strong feelings such as anger, fear, or anxiety before an injuring event.

- These feelings build, and the person has no way to express or address them directly.

Cutting or other self-injury provides a sense of relief; a release of the mounting tension.

- A feeling of guilt and shame usually follows the event.

- The feelings of shame paradoxically lead to continued self-injurious behavior.

The next time a similar strong feeling arises, the person has been "conditioned" to seek relief in the same way.

- The person feels compelled to repeat self-harm, which is likely to increase in frequency and degree.

- The person hides the tools used to injure, and covers up the evidence, often by wearing long sleeves.

Endorphins, specifically enkephalins, contribute to the "addictive" nature of self-injury.

- When a person injures themselves endorphins are released in the body and function as natural pain killers.

- The behavior may become addictive because the person learns to associate the act of self-injury with the positive feelings they get when endorphins are released in their system.

- The use of SSRI medications (selective serotonin reuptake inhibitors) such as Prozac and Zoloft, may be helpful in increasing brain serotonin levels and reducing self-injury in cases of moderate to severe depression.

❖ It's A Fact!!
FDA Suicide Warning

The U.S. Food and Drug Administration (FDA) requires that all antidepressant medications include a warning label about the increased risk of suicide in children, teens, and young adults. Young people should also be monitored for the emergence of agitation, irritability, and unusual changes in behavior, as these symptoms can indicate that the depression is getting worse. The risk of suicide is particularly great during the first one to two months of treatment.

Self-Injury And Suicide

Self-injury is usually not suicidal behavior but rather a way to reduce tensions. Inflicting physical harm on oneself is a poorly learned coping mechanism which is used to communicate feelings and self-soothe. Self-injury is strongly linked to a poor sense of self-worth, and over time, that depressed feeling can spiral into a suicidal attempt. Sometimes self-harm may accidentally go farther than intended, and a life-threatening injury may result, which is why intervention and profession help is required sooner rather than later.

Helping A Friend Or Family Member Who Is A Self-Injurer

No matter how you look at it, self-harm scares people. It is very hard coming to terms with the fact that someone you care about is physically harming themselves. From the depths of your own fear and helplessness you may feel frustrated if you are unable to get the person to stop hurting themselves which can further drive the person away.

Some Helpful Tips In Dealing With Someone Who Self-Injures

- Understand that self-harming behavior is an attempt to maintain a certain amount of control which in and of itself is a way of self-soothing.

- Let the person know that you care about them and are available to listen.

- Encourage expressions of emotions including anger.

- Spend time doing enjoyable activities together.

- Offer to help them find a therapist or support group.

- Don't make judgmental comments or tell the person to stop the self-harming behavior—people who feel worthless and powerless are even more likely to self-injure.

- If a child is self-injuring, prepare to address the difficulties in the family. Start with expressing feelings which is a common factor in self-injury—this is not about blame, but rather about learning new ways of dealing with family interactions and communications which can help the entire family.

How Can A Self-Injuring Person Stop This Behavior?

Self-injury is a behavior that over time becomes compulsive and addictive. Like any other addiction, even though other people think the person should stop, most addicts have a hard time just saying no to their behavior—even when they realize it is unhealthy.

What You Can Do To Help Yourself

- Acknowledge this is a problem. You are probably hurting on the inside and need professional help to stop this addictive behavior.

- Realize this is not about being a bad person. This is about recognizing that a behavior that helped you handle your feelings has become a big problem.

- Find one person you trust and get professional help. Maybe a friend, teacher, rabbi, minister, counselor, or relative. Tell them you need to talk about something serious that is bothering you.

- Get help in identifying what "triggers" your self-harming behaviors. Ask for help in developing ways to either avoid or address those triggers.

- Recognize that self-injury is an attempt to self-soothe. Learn how to develop better ways to calm and soothe yourself.

- Figure out what function the self-injury is serving. Replace the act of self-harm with learning how to express anger, sadness, and fear in healthy ways.

Treatments For Self-Injury

One danger connected with self-injury is that it tends to become an addictive behavior, a habit that is difficult to break even when the individual wants to stop. As with other addictions, qualified professional help is almost always necessary. It is important to find a therapist who understands this behavior and is not upset or repulsed by it. Call your doctor or insurance company for a referral to a mental health professional who specializes in self-injury.

- Cognitive-behavioral therapy may be used to help the person learn to recognize and address triggering feelings in healthier ways.

✔ Quick Tip
Alternatives To Avoid Self-Harm

- If you self-injure to deal with anger that you cannot express openly, try working through those feelings by doing something different: Running, dancing fast, screaming, punching a pillow, throwing something, ripping something apart.

- If you hurt yourself in order to feel something when you feel numb inside: Hold ice cubes in one hand and try to crush them, hold a package of frozen food, take a very cold shower, chew something with a very strong taste (like chili peppers, raw ginger root, or a grapefruit peel), wear an elastic rubber band around your wrist and snap it (in moderation to avoid bruising) when you feel like hurting yourself.

- If you inflict physical pain to calm yourself: Try taking a bubble bath, doing deep breathing, writing in a journal, drawing, or doing some yoga.

- If you self-mutilate to see blood: Try drawing a red ink line where you would usually cut yourself, in combination with the other suggestions above.

- Because a history of abuse or incest may be at the core of an individual's self-injuring behavior, therapies that address post-traumatic stress disorder such as eye movement desensitization and reprocessing (EMDR) may be helpful (visit Helpguide's website at www.helpguide.org for more information).

- Hypnosis or other self-relaxation techniques are helpful in reducing the stress and tension that often precede injuring incidents (Helpguide's website offers an article on Yoga, meditation, and other relaxation techniques).

- Group therapy may be helpful in decreasing the shame associated with self-harm and help to support healthy expressions of emotions.

- Family therapy may be useful, both in addressing any history of family stress related to the behavior and also in helping other family members learn how to communicate more directly and non-judgmentally with each other.

- In cases of moderate to severe depression or anxiety, an antidepressant or anti-anxiety medication may be used to reduce the impulsive urges to self-harm in response to stress, while other coping strategies are developed.

- In severe cases an in-patient hospitalization program with a multidisciplinary team approach may be required.

Chapter 18

Eating Disorders

Eating disorders are so common in America that one or two out of every 100 students will struggle with one.

Eating disorders are more than just going on a diet to lose weight or trying to make sure you exercise every day. They're extremes in eating behavior—the diet that never ends and gradually gets more restrictive, for example. Or the person who can't go out with friends because he or she thinks it's more important to go running to work off a piece of candy.

The most common types of eating disorder are anorexia nervosa and bulimia nervosa (usually called simply "anorexia" and "bulimia"). But other food-related disorders, like binge eating disorders, body image disorders, and food phobias, are showing up more frequently than they used to.

Anorexia

People with anorexia have an extreme fear of weight gain and a distorted view of their body size and shape. As a result, they can't maintain a normal body weight. Some people with anorexia restrict their food intake by dieting, fasting, or excessive exercise. They hardly eat at all—and the small amount of food they do eat becomes an obsession.

About This Chapter: "Eating Disorders," November 2007, reprinted with permission from www.kidshealth.org. Copyright © 2007 The Nemours Foundation. This information was provided by KidsHealth, one of the largest resources online for medically reviewed health information written for parents, kids, and teens. For more articles like this one, visit www.KidsHealth.org, or www.TeensHealth.org.

Other people with anorexia do something called binge eating and purging, where they eat a lot of food and then try to get rid of the calories by forcing themselves to vomit, using laxatives, or exercising excessively.

Bulimia

Bulimia is similar to anorexia. With bulimia, a person binge eats (eats a lot of food) and then tries to compensate in extreme ways, such as forced vomiting or excessive exercise, to prevent weight gain. Over time, these steps can be dangerous.

To be diagnosed with bulimia, a person must be binging and purging regularly, at least twice a week for a couple of months. Binge eating is different from going to a party and "pigging out" on pizza, then deciding to go to the gym the next day and eat more healthfully. People with bulimia eat a large amount of food (often junk food) at once, usually in secret. The person typically feels powerless to stop the eating and can only stop once he or she is too full to eat any more. Most people with bulimia then purge by vomiting, but may also use laxatives or excessive exercise.

Although anorexia and bulimia are very similar, people with anorexia are usually very thin and underweight but those with bulimia may be a normal weight or even overweight.

Binge Eating Disorder

This eating disorder is similar to anorexia and bulimia because a person binges regularly on food (more than three times a week). But, unlike the other eating disorders, a person with binge eating disorder does not try to "compensate" by purging the food.

Anorexia, bulimia, and binge eating disorder all involve unhealthy eating patterns that begin gradually and build to the point where a person feels unable to control them.

Anorexia And Bulimia: What To Look For

Sometimes a person with anorexia or bulimia starts out just trying to lose some weight or hoping to get in shape. But the urge to eat less or to purge spirals out of control.

❖ **It's A Fact!!**

Not Just A Girl Thing

More guys are seeking help for eating disorders. Guys with eating disorders tend to focus more on athletic appearance or success than on just looking thin.

People with anorexia or bulimia frequently have an intense fear of being fat or think that they are fat when they are not. A person with anorexia may weigh food before eating it or compulsively count the calories of everything. When it seems "normal" or "cool" to do things like restrict food intake to an unhealthy level, it's a sign that a person has a problem.

So how do you know if a person is struggling with anorexia or bulimia? You can't tell just by looking at someone. A person who loses a lot of weight may have another health condition or may be losing weight through healthy eating and exercise.

Here are some signs that a person may have anorexia or bulimia:

Anorexia

- Becomes very thin, frail, or emaciated
- Obsessed with eating, food, and weight control
- Weighs herself or himself repeatedly
- Counts or portions food carefully
- Only eats certain foods, avoiding foods like dairy, meat, wheat, etc. (of course, lots of people who are allergic to a particular food or are vegetarians avoid certain foods)
- Exercises excessively
- Feels fat
- Withdraws from social activities, especially meals and celebrations involving food may be depressed, lethargic (lacking in energy), and feel cold a lot

Bulimia

- Fears weight gain
- Intensely unhappy with body size, shape, and weight

- Makes excuses to go to the bathroom immediately after meals
- May only eat diet or low-fat foods (except during binges)
- Regularly buys laxatives, diuretics, or enemas
- Spends most of his or her time working out or trying to work off calories
- Withdraws from social activities, especially meals and celebrations involving food

What Causes Eating Disorders?

No one is really sure what causes eating disorders, although there are many theories about why people develop them. Many people who develop an eating disorder are between 13 and 17 years old. This is a time of emotional and physical changes, academic pressures, and a greater degree of peer pressure. Although there is a sense of greater independence during the teen years, teens might feel that they are not in control of their personal freedom and, sometimes, of their bodies. This can be especially true during puberty.

For girls, even though it's completely normal (and necessary) to gain some additional body fat during puberty, some respond to this change by becoming very fearful of their new weight. They might mistakenly feel compelled to get rid of it any way they can.

When you combine the pressure to be like celeb role models with the fact that during puberty our bodies change, it's not hard to see why some teens develop a negative view of themselves.

✤ It's A Fact!!
A Not-So-Perfect Picture

We're overloaded by images of thin celebrities—people who often weigh far less than their healthy weight (and who may have histories of eating disorders). So it's easy to see why people may develop a fear of weight gain, even if that weight gain is temporary and healthy.

Many people with eating disorders also can be depressed or anxious, or have other mental health problems such as obsessive-compulsive disorder (OCD). There is also evidence that eating disorders may run in families. Although part of this may be our in genes, it's also because we learn our values and behaviors from our families.

Sports And Eating Disorders

Athletes and dancers are particularly vulnerable to developing eating disorders around the time of puberty, as they may want to stop or suppress growth (both height and weight).

Coaches, family members, and others may encourage teens in certain sports—such as gymnastics, ice-skating, and ballet—to be as thin as possible. Some athletes and runners are also encouraged to weigh less or shed body fat at a time when they are biologically destined to gain it.

Effects Of Eating Disorders

Eating disorders are serious medical illnesses. They often go along with other problems such as stress, anxiety, depression, and substance use. People with eating disorders also can have serious physical health problems, such as heart conditions or kidney failure. People who weigh at least 15% less than the normal weight for their height may not have enough body fat to keep their organs and other body parts healthy. In severe cases, eating disorders can lead to severe malnutrition and even death.

With anorexia, the body goes into starvation mode, and the lack of nutrition can affect the body in many ways:

- A drop in blood pressure, pulse, and breathing rate
- Hair loss and fingernail breakage
- Loss of periods
- Lanugo hair—a soft hair that can grow all over the skin
- Lightheadedness and inability to concentrate
- Anemia

- Swollen joints
- Brittle bones

With bulimia, constant vomiting and lack of nutrients can cause these problems:

- Constant stomach pain
- Damage to a person's stomach and kidneys
- Tooth decay (from exposure to stomach acids)
- "Chipmunk cheeks," when the salivary glands permanently expand from throwing up so often
- Loss of periods
- Loss of the mineral potassium (this can contribute to heart problems and even death)

A person with binge eating disorder who gains a lot of weight is at risk of developing diabetes, heart disease, and some of the other diseases associated with being overweight.

The emotional pain of an eating disorder can take its toll, too. When a person becomes obsessed with weight, it's hard to concentrate on much else. Many people with eating disorders become withdrawn and less social. People with eating disorders might not join in on snacks and meals with their friends or families, and they often don't want to break from their intense exercise routine to have fun.

People with eating disorders often spend a lot of mental energy on planning what they eat, how to avoid food, or their next binge, spend a lot of their money on food, hide in the bathroom for a long time after meals, or make excuses for going on long walks (alone) after a meal.

Treatment For Eating Disorders

Fortunately, people with eating disorders can get well and gradually learn to eat normally again. Eating disorders involve both the mind and body. So medical doctors, mental health professionals, and dietitians will often be involved in a person's treatment and recovery.

Therapy or counseling is a critical part of treating eating disorders—in many cases, family therapy is one of the keys to eating healthily again. Parents and other family members are important in helping a person see that his or her normal body shape is perfectly fine and that being excessively thin can be dangerous.

If you want to talk to someone about eating disorders and you don't feel as though you can approach a parent, try talking to a teacher, a neighbor, your doctor, or another trusted adult. Remember that eating disorders are very common among teens. Treatment options depend on each person and their families, but many options are available to help you overcome an eating disorder. Therapy can help you feel in charge again and learn to like your body, just as it is.

☞ Remember!!
Don't Wait To Get Help

Like all bad habits, unhealthy eating patterns become harder to break the longer a person does them. The most critical thing about treating eating disorders is to recognize and address the problem as soon as possible. Eating disorders can do a lot of damage to the body and mind if left untreated, and they don't get better by themselves.

Part Three

Recognizing And Treating Suicidal Ideation

Chapter 19

If You Are Considering Suicide...
Read This First

The last thing that most people expect is that they will run out of reasons to live. But if you are experiencing suicidal thoughts, you need to know that you're not alone. By some estimates, as many as one in six people will become seriously suicidal at some point in their lives.

Some Important Facts The American Association Of Suicidology Would Like To Share With You

Suicidal thinking is usually associated with problems that can be treated.

Clinical depression, anxiety disorders, chemical dependency, and other disorders produce profound emotional distress. They also interfere with effective problem-solving. But you need to know that studies show that the vast majority of people who receive appropriate treatment improve or recover completely. Even if you have received treatment before, you should know that different treatments work better for different people in different situations. Several tries are sometimes necessary before the right combination is found.

If you are unable to think of solutions other than suicide, it is not that solutions don't exist, only that you are currently unable to see them.

About This Chapter: "If You Are Considering Suicide," © 2009 American Association of Suicidology (www.suicidology.org). Reprinted with permission.

Therapists and counselors (and sometimes friends) can help you to see solutions that otherwise are not apparent to you.

Suicidal Crises Are Almost Always Temporary

Although it might seem as if your unhappiness will never end, it is important to realize that crises are usually time-limited. Solutions are found, feelings change, unexpected positive events occur. Suicide is sometimes referred to as "a permanent solution to a temporary problem." Don't let suicide rob you of better times that will come your way when you allow more time to pass.

Problems Are Seldom As Great As They Appear At First Glance

Job loss, financial problems, loss of important people in our lives—all such stressful events can seem catastrophic at the time they are happening. Then, month or years later, they usually look smaller and more manageable. Sometimes, imagining ourselves "five years down the road" can help us to see that a problem that currently seems catastrophic will pass and that we will survive.

☞ Remember!!
Do Not Keep Suicidal Thoughts To Yourself

Help is available for you, whether through a friend, therapist, or member of the clergy. Find someone you trust and let them know how bad things are. This can be your first step on the road to healing.

Telephone Numbers For More Information On Receiving Help

National Mental Health Association 703-684-7722

Anxiety Disorders Association of America 301-231-9350

American Psychological Association 202-336-5500

American Psychiatric Association 202-682-6000

Depressive and Manic-Depressive Association 312-642-0049

National Alliance for the Mentally Ill 703-524-7600

National Suicide Prevention Lifeline 800-273-TALK (8255)

Reasons For Living Can Help Sustain A Person In Pain

A famous psychologist once conducted a study of Nazi concentration camp survivors, and found that those who survived almost always reported strong beliefs about what was important in life. You, too, might be able to strengthen your connection with life if you consider what has sustained you through hard times in the past. Family ties, religion, love of art or nature, and dreams for the future are just a few of the many aspects of life that provide meaning and gratification, but which we can lose sight of due to emotional distress.

Chapter 20

My Friend Is Talking About Suicide

Warning Signs Of Suicide

Everyone feels sad, depressed, or angry sometimes—especially when the pressures of school, friends, and family become too much to handle. Other times, though, feelings of sadness or hopelessness just won't go away. These feelings may begin to affect many areas of a person's life and outlook. Someone who experiences very intense feelings of depression or irritability may begin to think about suicide.

You may have heard that people who talk about suicide won't actually go through with it. That's not true. People who talk about suicide may be likely to try it.

Other warning signs that someone may be thinking of suicide include:

• talking about suicide or death in general;

• talking about "going away";

• talking about feeling hopeless or feeling guilty;

About This Chapter: "My Friend Is Talking About Suicide," June 2008, reprinted with permission from www.kidshealth.org. Copyright © 2008 The Nemours Foundation. This information was provided by KidsHealth, one of the largest resources online for medically reviewed health information written for parents, kids, and teens. For more articles like this one, visit www.KidsHealth.org, or www.TeensHealth.org.

- pulling away from friends or family and losing the desire to go out;

- having no desire to take part in favorite activities;

- having trouble concentrating or thinking clearly;

- experiencing changes in eating or sleeping habits;

- engaging in self-destructive behavior (drinking alcohol, taking drugs, or driving too fast, for example).

✤ It's A Fact!!
Why Is Suicide A
Public Health Problem?

- More than 33,000 people kill themselves each year.

- More than 395,000 people with self-inflicted injuries are treated in emergency rooms each year.

Source: From "Understanding Suicide," Centers for Disease Control and Prevention, 2009.

As a friend, you may also know if the person is going through some tough times. Sometimes, a specific event, stress, or crisis—like a relationship breaking up or a death in the family—can trigger suicidal behavior in someone who is already feeling depressed and showing the warning signs listed above.

What You Can Do

Ask

If you have a friend who is talking about suicide or showing other warning signs, don't wait to see if he or she starts to feel better. Talk about it. Most of the time, people who are considering suicide are willing to discuss it if someone asks them out of concern and care.

Some people (both teens and adults) are reluctant to ask teens if they have been thinking about suicide or hurting themselves. That's because they're afraid that, by asking, they may plant the idea of suicide. This is not true. It is always a good thing to ask.

Starting the conversation with someone you think may be considering suicide helps in many ways. First, it allows you to get help for the person. Second, just talking about it may help the person to feel less alone, less isolated, and more cared about and understood—the opposite of the feelings that may have led to suicidal thinking to begin with. Third, talking may provide a chance to consider that there may be another solution.

Asking someone if he or she is having thoughts about suicide can be difficult. Sometimes it helps to let your friend know why you are asking. For instance, you might say, "I've noticed that you've been talking a lot about wanting to be dead. Have you been having thoughts about trying to kill yourself?"

Listen

Listen to your friend without judging and offer reassurance that you're there and you care. If you think your friend is in immediate danger, stay close—make sure he or she isn't left alone.

Tell

Even if you're sworn to secrecy and you feel like you'll be betraying your friend if you tell, you should still seek help. Share your concerns with an adult you trust as soon as possible. If necessary, you can also call a local emergency number (911) or the toll-free number for a suicide crisis line (you can find local suicide crisis numbers listed in your phone book).

The important thing is to notify a responsible adult. Although it may be tempting to try to help your friend on your own, it's always safest to get help.

After Suicide

Sometimes even if you get help and adults intervene, a friend or classmate may attempt or die by suicide. When this happens, it's common to have many different emotions. Some teens say they feel guilty—especially if they felt they could have interpreted their friend's actions and words better. Others say they feel angry with the person for doing something so selfish. Still others say they feel nothing at all—they are too filled with grief.

When someone attempts suicide, those who know that person may feel afraid or uncomfortable about talking to him or her. Try to overcome these feelings of discomfort—this is a time when someone absolutely needs to feel connected to others.

If you are having difficulty dealing with a friend or classmate's suicide, it's best to talk to an adult you trust. Feeling grief after a friend dies by suicide is normal. But if that sadness begins to interfere with your everyday life, it's a sign that you may need to speak with someone about your feelings.

🕮☞ Remember!!
Who is at risk for suicide?

Suicide affects everyone, but some groups are at higher risk than others. Men are four times more likely than women to die from suicide. However, three times more women than men report attempting suicide. In addition, suicide rates are high among middle aged and older adults.

Several factors can put a person at risk for attempting or committing suicide. But, having these risk factors does not always mean that suicide will occur.

Risk factors for suicide include the following:

- Previous suicide attempt(s)
- History of depression or other mental illness
- Alcohol or drug abuse
- Family history of suicide or violence
- Physical illness
- Feeling alone

Source: From "Understanding Suicide," Centers for Disease Control and Prevention, 2009.

Chapter 21

Why Does A Person Consider Suicide?

Suicide

Ethan felt like there was no point going on with life. Things had been tough since his mom died. His dad was working two jobs and seemed frazzled and angry most of the time. Whenever he and Ethan talked, it usually ended in yelling.

Ethan had just found out he'd failed a math test, and he was afraid of how mad and disappointed his dad would be. In the past, he always talked things over with his girlfriend—the only person who seemed to understand. But they'd broken up the week before, and now Ethan felt he had nowhere to turn.

Ethan knew where his dad kept his guns. But as he was unlocking the cabinet, he heard his kid sister arriving home from school. He didn't want Grace to be the person to find him, so he put the gun back and went to watch TV with her instead. Later, when he realized how close he'd come to ending his life, Ethan was terrified. He summoned the courage to talk to his dad. After a long conversation, he realized how much his dad cared. All he could think of was how he'd almost thrown it all away.

About This Chapter: "Suicide," June 2008, reprinted with permission from www.kidshealth. org. Copyright © 2008 The Nemours Foundation. This information was provided by KidsHealth, one of the largest resources online for medically reviewed health information written for parents, kids, and teens. For more articles like this one, visit www.KidsHealth .org, or www.TeensHealth.org.

Why Do Teens Try To Kill Themselves?

Most teens interviewed after making a suicide attempt say that they did it because they were trying to escape from a situation that seemed impossible to deal with or to get relief from really bad thoughts or feelings. Like Ethan, they didn't want to die as much as they wanted to escape from what was going on. And at that particular moment dying seemed like the only way out.

Some people who end their lives or attempt suicide might be trying to escape feelings of rejection, hurt, or loss. Others might be angry, ashamed, or guilty about something. Some people may be worried about disappointing friends or family members. And some may feel unwanted, unloved, victimized, or like they're a burden to others.

We all feel overwhelmed by difficult emotions or situations sometimes. But most people get through it or can put their problems in perspective and find a way to carry on with determination and hope. So why does one person try suicide when another person in the same tough situation does not? What makes some people more resilient (better able to deal with life's setbacks and difficulties) than others? What makes a person unable to see another way out of a bad situation besides ending his or her life?

The answer to those questions lies in the fact that most people who commit suicide have depression.

Depression

Depression leads people to focus mostly on failures and disappointments, to emphasize the negative side of their situations, and to downplay their own capabilities or worth. Someone with severe depression is unable to see the possibility of a good outcome and may believe they will never be happy or things will never go right for them again.

Depression affects a person's thoughts in such a way that the person doesn't see when a problem can be overcome. It's as if the depression puts a filter on the person's thinking that distorts things. That's why depressed people don't realize that suicide is a permanent solution to a temporary problem in the same way that other people do. A teen with depression may feel like there's no other way out of problems, no other escape from emotional pain, or no other way to communicate their desperate unhappiness.

> ❖ **It's A Fact!!**
> Unfortunately teen are vulnerable to depression. That's because hormones and sleep cycles, which both change dramatically during adolescence, can affect mood. The good news is that depression is treatable. Most teens get better with the right help.

Sometimes people who feel suicidal may not even realize they are depressed. They are unaware that it is the depression — not the situation — that's influencing them to see things in a "there's no way out," "it will never get better," "there's nothing I can do" kind of way.

When depression lifts because a person gets the proper therapy or treatment, the distorted thinking is cleared. The person can find pleasure, energy, and hope again. But while someone is seriously depressed, suicidal thinking is a real concern.

People with a condition called bipolar disorder are also more at risk for suicide because their condition can cause them to go through times when they are extremely depressed as well as times when they have abnormally high or frantic energy (called mania or manic). Both of these extreme phases of bipolar disorder affect and distort a person's mood, outlook, and judgment. For people with this condition, it can be a challenge to keep problems in perspective and act with good judgment.

Substance Abuse

Teens with alcohol and drug problems are also more at risk for suicidal thinking and behavior. Alcohol and some drugs have depressive effects on the brain. Misuse of these substances can bring on serious depression. That's especially true for some teens who already have a tendency to depression because of their biology, family history, or other life stressors.

The problem can be made worse because many people who are depressed turn to alcohol or drugs as an escape. But they may not realize that the depressive effects alcohol and drugs have on the brain can actually intensify depression in the long run.

In addition to their depressive effects, alcohol and drugs alter a person's judgment. They interfere with the ability to assess risk, make good choices, and think of solutions to problems. Many suicide attempts occur when a person is under the influence of alcohol or drugs.

This doesn't mean that everyone who is depressed or who has an alcohol or drug problem will try to kill themselves, of course. But these conditions—especially both together—increase a person's risk for suicide.

Suicide Is Not Always Planned

Sometimes a depressed person plans a suicide in advance. Many times, though, suicide attempts happen impulsively, in a moment of feeling desperately upset. A situation like a breakup, a big fight with a parent, an unintended pregnancy, being outed by someone else, or being victimized in any way can cause someone to feel desperately upset. Often, a situation like this, on top of an existing depression, acts like the final straw.

Some people who attempt suicide mean to die and some aren't completely sure they want to die. For some, a suicide attempt is a way to express deep emotional pain. They can't say how they feel, so, for them, attempting suicide feels like the only way to get their message across. Sadly, many people who really didn't mean to kill themselves end up dead or critically ill.

Warning Signs

There are often signs that someone may be thinking about or planning a suicide attempt. Here are some of them:

- Talking about suicide or death in general

- Talking about "going away"

- Referring to things they "won't be needing," and giving away possessions

- Talking about feeling hopeless or feeling guilty

- Pulling away from friends or family and losing the desire to go out

- Having no desire to take part in favorite things or activities

- Having trouble concentrating or thinking clearly

- Experiencing changes in eating or sleeping habits

- Engaging in self-destructive behavior (drinking alcohol, taking drugs, or cutting, for example)

What If This Is You?

If you have been thinking about suicide, get help now. Depression is powerful. You can't wait and hope that your mood might improve. When a person has been feeling down for a long time, it's hard to step back and be objective.

Talk to someone you trust as soon as you can. If you can't talk to a parent, talk to a coach, a relative, a school counselor, a religious leader, or a teacher. Call a suicide crisis line (such as 1-800-SUICIDE or 1-800-999-9999) or your local emergency number (911). These toll-free lines are staffed 24 hours a day, seven days a week by trained professionals who can help you without ever knowing your name or seeing your face. All calls are confidential—no one you know will find out that you've called. They are there to help you figure out how to work through tough situations.

What If It's Someone You Know?

It is always a good thing to start a conversation with someone you think may be considering suicide. It allows you to get help for the person, and just talking about it may help the person to feel less alone and more cared about and understood.

Talking things through may also give the person an opportunity to consider other solutions to problems. Most of the time, people who are considering suicide are willing to talk if someone asks them out of concern and care. Because people who are depressed are not as able to see answers as well as others, it can help to have someone work with them in coming up with at least one other way out of a bad situation.

❖ It's A Fact!!

Girls attempt suicide more often than guys, but guys are about four times more likely to succeed when they try to kill themselves. This is because guys tend to use more deadly methods, like guns or hanging. More than half of all suicide deaths involve a gun.

Even if a friend or classmate swears you to secrecy, you must get help as soon as possible—your friend's life could depend on it. Someone who is seriously thinking about suicide may have sunk so deeply into an emotional hole that the person could be unable to recognize that he or she needs help. Tell an adult you trust as soon as possible.

If necessary, you can also call the toll-free number for a suicide crisis line or a local emergency number (911). You can find local suicide crisis or hotline numbers listed in your phone book. These are confidential resources and the people at any of these places are happy to talk to you to help you figure out what is best to do.

Sometimes, teens who make a suicide attempt—or who die as a result of suicide—seem to give no clue beforehand. This can leave loved ones feeling not only grief stricken but guilty and wondering if they missed something. It is important for family members and friends of those who die by suicide to know that sometimes there is no warning and they should not blame themselves.

When someone dies by suicide the people left behind can wrestle with a terrible emotional pain. Teens who have had a recent loss or crisis or who had a family member or classmate who committed suicide may be especially vulnerable to suicidal thinking and behavior themselves.

If you've been close to someone who has attempted or committed suicide, it can help to talk with a therapist or counselor—someone who is trained in dealing with this complex issue. Or, you could join a group for survivors where you can share your feelings and get the support of people who have been in the same situation as you.

Coping With Problems

Being a teen is not easy. There are many new social, academic, and personal pressures. And for teens who have additional problems to deal with, such as living in violent or abusive environments, life can feel even more difficult.

Some teens worry about sexuality and relationships, wondering if their feelings and attractions are normal, or if they will be loved and accepted. Others struggle with body image and eating problems; trying to reach an impossible ideal leaves them feeling bad about themselves. Some teens have learning problems or attention problems that make it hard for them to succeed in school. They may feel disappointed in themselves or feel they are a disappointment to others.

These problems can be difficult and draining—and can lead to depression if they go on too long without relief or support. We all struggle with painful problems and events at times. How do people get through it without becoming depressed? Part of it is staying connected to family, friends, school, faith, and other support networks. People are better able to deal with tough circumstances when they have at least one person who believes in them, wants the best for them, and in whom they can confide. People also cope better when they keep in mind that most problems are temporary and can be overcome.

When struggling with problems, it helps to:

- Tell someone you trust what's going on with you.
- Be around people who are caring and positive.
- Ask someone to help you figure out what to do about a problem you're facing.
- Work with a therapist or counselor if problems are getting you down and depressed—or if you don't have a strong support network, or feel you can't cope.

Counselors and therapists can provide emotional support and can help teens build their own coping skills for dealing with problems. It can also help to join a support network for people who are going through the same problems—for example, anorexia and body image issues, living with an alcoholic family member, or sexuality and sexual health concerns. These groups can help provide a caring environment where you can talk through problems with people who share your concerns.

Check out your phone book to find local support groups, or ask a school counselor or a youth group leader to help you find what you need.

🖝 Remember!!

Suicide attempts are highest during middle adolescence. By about age 17 or 18, the rate of suicide attempts drops. This may be because older teens have learned to tolerate sad or upset moods, know how to get the support they need, and have developed better coping skills.

Chapter 22

How Can Psychotherapy Help?

What Is Psychotherapy?

Psychotherapy, or "talk therapy," is a way to treat people with a mental disorder by helping them understand their illness. It teaches people strategies and gives them tools to deal with stress and unhealthy thoughts and behaviors. Psychotherapy helps patients manage their symptoms better and function at their best in everyday life.

What Are The Different Types Of Psychotherapy?

Many kinds of psychotherapy exist. There is no "one-size-fits-all" approach. In addition, some therapies have been scientifically tested more than others. Some people may have a treatment plan that includes only one type of psychotherapy. Others receive treatment that includes elements of several different types. The kind of psychotherapy a person receives depends on his or her needs.

This section explains several of the most commonly used psychotherapies. However, it does not cover every detail about psychotherapy. Patients should talk to their doctor or a psychotherapist about planning treatment that meets their needs.

About This Chapter: This chapter includes text from "Psychotherapies," National Institute of Mental Health (www.nimh.nih.gov), 2009. The complete text of this document, including references, can be found online at http://www.nimh.nih.gov/health/topics/psychotherapies/index.shtml.

☞ Remember!!

Sometimes psychotherapy alone may be the best treatment for a person, depending on the illness and its severity. Other times, psychotherapy is combined with medications. Therapists work with an individual or families to devise an appropriate treatment plan.

Cognitive Behavioral Therapy

Cognitive behavioral therapy (CBT) is a blend of two therapies: cognitive therapy (CT) and behavioral therapy. CT was developed by psychotherapist Aaron Beck, MD, in the 1960s. CT focuses on a person's thoughts and beliefs, and how they influence a person's mood and actions, and aims to change a person's thinking to be more adaptive and healthy. Behavioral therapy focuses on a person's actions and aims to change unhealthy behavior patterns.

CBT helps a person focus on his or her current problems and how to solve them. Both patient and therapist need to be actively involved in this process. The therapist helps the patient learn how to identify distorted or unhelpful thinking patterns, recognize and change inaccurate beliefs, relate to others in more positive ways, and change behaviors accordingly.

CBT can be applied and adapted to treat many specific mental disorders.

CBT For Depression: Many studies have shown that CBT is a particularly effective treatment for depression, especially minor or moderate depression. Some people with depression may be successfully treated with CBT only. Others may need both CBT and medication. CBT helps people with depression restructure negative thought patterns. Doing so helps people interpret their environment and interactions with others in a positive and realistic way. It may also help a person recognize things that may be contributing to the depression and help him or her change behaviors that may be making the depression worse.

CBT For Anxiety Disorders: CBT for anxiety disorders aims to help a person develop a more adaptive response to a fear. A CBT therapist may use "exposure" therapy to treat certain anxiety disorders, such as a specific phobia, post traumatic stress disorder, or obsessive compulsive disorder. Exposure therapy has been found to be effective in treating anxiety-related disorders. It works by helping a person confront a specific fear or memory while in a safe and supportive environment. The main goals of exposure therapy are to help the patient learn that anxiety can lessen over time and give him or her the tools to cope with fear or traumatic memories.

A recent study sponsored by the Centers for Disease Control and Prevention concluded that CBT is effective in treating trauma-related disorders in children and teens.

CBT For Bipolar Disorder: People with bipolar disorder usually need to take medication, such as a mood stabilizer. But CBT is often used as an added treatment. The medication can help stabilize a person's mood so that he or she is receptive to psychotherapy and can get the most out of it. CBT can help a person cope with bipolar symptoms and learn to recognize when a mood shift is about to occur. CBT also helps a person with bipolar disorder stick with a treatment plan to reduce the chances of relapse (for example, when symptoms return).

CBT For Eating Disorders: Eating disorders can be very difficult to treat. However, some small studies have found that CBT can help reduce the risk of relapse in adults with anorexia who have restored their weight. CBT may also reduce some symptoms of bulimia, and it may also help some people reduce binge-eating behavior.

CBT For Schizophrenia: Treating schizophrenia with CBT is challenging. The disorder usually requires medication first. But research has shown that CBT, as an add-on to medication, can help a patient cope with schizophrenia. CBT helps patients learn more adaptive and realistic interpretations of events. Patients are also taught various coping techniques for dealing with "voices" or other hallucinations. They learn how to identify what triggers episodes of the illness, which can prevent or reduce the chances of relapse.

CBT for schizophrenia also stresses skill-oriented therapies. Patients learn skills to cope with life's challenges. The therapist teaches social, daily functioning, and problem-solving skills. This can help patients with schizophrenia minimize the types of stress that can lead to outbursts and hospitalizations.

Dialectical Behavior Therapy

Dialectical behavior therapy (DBT), a form of CBT, was developed by Marsha Linehan, PhD. At first, it was developed to treat people with suicidal thoughts and actions. It is now also used to treat people with borderline personality disorder (BPD). BPD is an illness in which suicidal thinking and actions are more common.

DBT emphasizes the value of a strong and equal relationship between patient and therapist. The therapist consistently reminds the patient when his or her behavior is unhealthy or disruptive—when boundaries are overstepped—and then teaches the skills needed to better deal with future similar situations. DBT involves both individual and group therapy. Individual sessions are used to teach new skills, while group sessions provide the opportunity to practice these skills.

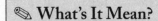 **What's It Mean?**

The term "dialectical" refers to a philosophic exercise in which two opposing views are discussed until a logical blending or balance of the two extremes—the middle way—is found. In keeping with that philosophy, the therapist assures the patient that the patient's behavior and feelings are valid and understandable. At the same time, the therapist coaches the patient to understand that it is his or her personal responsibility to change unhealthy or disruptive behavior.

Research suggests that DBT is an effective treatment for people with BPD. A recent study funded by the National Institute of Mental Health (NIMH) found that DBT reduced suicide attempts by half compared to other types of treatment for patients with BPD.

Interpersonal Therapy

Interpersonal therapy (IPT) is most often used on a one-on-one basis to treat depression or dysthymia (a more persistent but less severe form of depression). The current manual-based form of IPT used today was developed in the 1980's by Gerald Klerman, MD, and Myrna Weissman, MD.

IPT is based on the idea that improving communication patterns and the ways people relate to others will effectively treat depression. IPT helps identify how a person interacts with other people. When a behavior is causing problems, IPT guides the person to change the behavior. IPT explores major issues that may add to a person's depression, such as grief, or times of upheaval or transition. Sometimes IPT is used along with antidepressant medications.

IPT varies depending on the needs of the patient and the relationship between the therapist and patient. Basically, a therapist using IPT helps the patient identify troubling emotions and their triggers. The therapist helps the patient learn to express appropriate emotions in a healthy way. The patient may also examine relationships in his or her past that may have been affected by distorted mood and behavior. Doing so can help the patient learn to be more objective about current relationships.

Studies vary as to the effectiveness of IPT. It may depend on the patient, the disorder, the severity of the disorder, and other variables. In general, however, IPT is found to be effective in treating depression.

A variation of IPT called interpersonal and social rhythm therapy (IPSRT) was developed to treat bipolar disorder. IPSRT combines the basic principles of IPT with behavioral psychoeducation designed to help patients adopt regular daily routines and sleep/wake cycles, stick with medication treatment, and improve relationships. Research has found that when IPSRT is combined with medication, it is an effective treatment for bipolar disorder. IPSRT is as effective as other types of psychotherapy combined with medication in helping to prevent a relapse of bipolar symptoms.

Family-Focused Therapy

Family-focused therapy (FFT) was developed by David Miklowitz, PhD, and Michael Goldstein, PhD, for treating bipolar disorder. It was designed with the assumption that a patient's relationship with his or her family is vital to the success of managing the illness. FFT includes family members in therapy sessions to improve family relationships, which may support better treatment results.

Therapists trained in FFT work to identify difficulties and conflicts among family members that may be worsening the patient's illness. Therapy is meant to help members find more effective ways to resolve those difficulties.

The therapist educates family members about their loved one's disorder, its symptoms and course, and how to help their relative manage it more effectively. When families learn about the disorder, they may be able to spot early signs of a relapse and create an action plan that involves all family members. During therapy, the therapist will help family members recognize when they express unhelpful criticism or hostility toward their relative with bipolar disorder. The therapist will teach family members how to communicate negative emotions in a better way. Several studies have found FFT to be effective in helping a patient become stabilized and preventing relapses.

FFT also focuses on the stress family members feel when they care for a relative with bipolar disorder. The therapy aims to prevent family members from "burning out" or disengaging from the effort. The therapist helps the family accept how bipolar disorder can limit their relative. At the same time,

---

✤ It's A Fact!!
Are psychotherapies different for children and adolescents?

Psychotherapies can be adapted to the needs of children and adolescents, depending on the mental disorder. For example, the NIMH-funded Treatment of Adolescents with Depression Study (TADS) found that CBT, when combined with antidepressant medication, was the most effective treatment over the short term for teens with major depression. CBT by itself was also an effective treatment, especially over the long term. Studies have found that individual and group-based CBT are effective treatments for child and adolescent anxiety disorders. Other studies have found that IPT is an effective treatment for child and adolescent depression.

Psychosocial treatments that involve a child's parents and family also have been shown to be effective, especially for disruptive disorders such as conduct disorder or oppositional defiant disorder. Some effective treatments are designed to reduce the child's problem behaviors and improve parent-child interactions. Focusing on behavioral parent management training, parents are taught the skills they need to encourage and reward positive behaviors in their children. Similar training helps parents manage their child's attention deficit/hyperactivity disorder (ADHD). This approach, which has been shown to be effective, can be combined with approaches directed at children to help them learn problem-solving, anger management and social interaction skills.

the therapist holds the patient responsible for his or her own well being and actions to a level that is appropriate for the person's age.

Generally, the family and patient attend sessions together. The needs of each patient and family are different, and those needs determine the exact course of treatment. However, the main components of a structured FFT usually include the following:

- Family education on bipolar disorder

- Building communication skills to better deal with stress

- Solving problems together as a family

It is important to acknowledge and address the needs of family members. Research has shown that primary caregivers of people with bipolar disorder

---

Family-based therapy may also be used to treat adolescents with eating disorders. One type is called the Maudsley approach, named after the Maudsley Hospital in London, where the approach was developed. This type of outpatient family therapy is used to treat anorexia nervosa in adolescents. It considers the active participation of parents to be essential in the recovery of their teen. The Maudsley approach proceeds through three phases:

- **Weight Restoration:** Parents become fully responsible for ensuring that their teen eats. A therapist helps parents better understand their teen's disease. Parents learn how to avoid criticizing their teen, but they also learn to make sure that their teen eats.

- **Returning Control Over Eating To The Teen:** Once the teen accepts the control parents have over his or her eating habits, parents may begin giving up that control. Parents are encouraged to help their teen take more control over eating again.

- **Establishing Healthy Adolescent Identity:** When the teen has reached and maintained a healthy weight, the therapist helps him or her begin developing a healthy sense of identity and autonomy.

Several studies have found the Maudsley approach to be successful in treating teens with anorexia. Currently a large-scale study funded by the National Institute of Mental Health (NIMH) on the approach is under way.

are at increased risk for illness themselves. For example, a 2007 study based on results from the NIMH-funded Systematic Treatment Enhancement Program for Bipolar Disorder (STEP-BD) trial found that primary caregivers of participants were at high risk for developing sleep problems and chronic conditions, such as high blood pressure. However, the caregivers were less likely to see a doctor for their own health issues. In addition, a 2005 study found that 33 percent of caregivers of bipolar patients had clinically significant levels of depression.

What Other Types Of Therapies Are Used?

In addition to the therapies listed above, many more approaches exist. Some types have been scientifically tested more than others. Also, some of these therapies are constantly evolving. They are often combined with more established psychotherapies. A few examples of other therapies are described here.

- **Psychodynamic Therapy:** Historically, psychodynamic therapy was tied to the principles of psychoanalytic theory, which asserts that a person's behavior is affected by his or her unconscious mind and past experiences. Now therapists who use psychodynamic therapy rarely include psychoanalytic methods. Rather, psychodynamic therapy helps people gain greater self-awareness and understanding about their own actions. It helps patients identify and explore how their nonconscious emotions and motivations can influence their behavior. Sometimes ideas from psychodynamic therapy are interwoven with other types of therapy, like CBT or IPT, to treat various types of mental disorders. Research on psychodynamic therapy is mixed. However, a review of 23 clinical trials involving psychodynamic therapy found it to be as effective as other established psychotherapies.

- **Light Therapy:** Light therapy is used to treat seasonal affective disorder (SAD), a form of depression that usually occurs during the autumn and winter months, when the amount of natural sunlight decreases. Scientists think SAD occurs in some people when their bodies' daily rhythms are upset by short days and long nights. Research has found that the hormone melatonin is affected by this seasonal change. Melatonin normally works to regulate the body's rhythms and responses to light and dark. During light therapy, a person sits in front of a "light box" for periods of time, usually in the morning. The box emits a full spectrum light, and sitting in front of it appears to help reset the body's daily rhythms. Also, some research indicates that a low dose of melatonin, taken at specific times of the day, can also help treat SAD.

Other types of therapies sometimes used in conjunction with the more established therapies include the following:

- **Expressive Or Creative Arts Therapy:** Expressive or creative arts therapy is based on the idea that people can help heal themselves through art, music, dance, writing, or other expressive acts. One study has found that expressive writing can reduce depression symptoms among women who were victims of domestic violence. It also helps college students at risk for depression.

- **Animal-Assisted Therapy:** Working with animals, such as horses, dogs, or cats, may help some people cope with trauma, develop empathy, and encourage better communication. Companion animals are sometimes introduced in hospitals, psychiatric wards, nursing homes, and other places where they may bring comfort and have a mild therapeutic effect. Animal-assisted therapy has also been used as an added therapy for children with mental disorders. Research on the approach is limited, but a recent study found it to be moderately effective in easing behavioral problems and promoting emotional well-being.

- **Play Therapy:** This therapy is used with children. It involves the use of toys and games to help a child identify and talk about his or her feelings, as well as establish communication with a therapist. A therapist can sometimes better understand a child's problems by watching how he or she plays. Research in play therapy is minimal.

Chapter 23

Going To A Therapist: What To Expect

Eric went to therapy a couple of years ago when his parents were getting divorced. Although he no longer goes, he feels the two months he spent in therapy helped him get through the tough times as his parents worked out their differences.

Melody began seeing her therapist a year ago when she was being bullied at school. She still goes every two weeks because she feels therapy is really helping to build her self-esteem.

Britt just joined a therapy group for eating disorders led by her school's psychologist, and her friend Dana said she'd go with her.

When our parents were in school, very few kids went to therapy. Now it's much more common and also more accepted. Lots of teens wonder if therapy could help them.

What Are Some Reasons That Teens Go To Therapists?

When teens are going through a rough time, such as family troubles or problems in school, they might feel more supported if they talk to a therapist. They may be feeling sad, angry, or overwhelmed by what's been happening—

About This Chapter: "Going To A Therapist," August 2007, reprinted with permission from www.kidshealth.org. Copyright © 2007 The Nemours Foundation. This information was provided by KidsHealth, one of the largest resources online for medically reviewed health information written for parents, kids, and teens. For more articles like this one, visit www.KidsHealth.org, or www.TeensHealth.org.

and need help sorting out their feelings, finding solutions to their problems, or just feeling better. That's when therapy can help.

Just a few examples of situations in which therapy can help are when someone:

- feels sad, depressed, worried, shy, or just stressed out;

- is dieting or overeating for too long or it becomes a problem (eating disorders);

- cuts, burns, or self-injures;

- is dealing with an attention problem (ADHD) or a learning problem;

- is coping with a chronic illness (such as diabetes or asthma) or a new diagnosis of a serious problem such as HIV, cancer, or a sexually transmitted disease (STD);

- is dealing with family changes such as separation and divorce, or family problems such as alcoholism or addiction;

- is trying to cope with a traumatic event, death of a loved one, or worry over world events;

- has a habit he or she would like to get rid of, such as nail biting, hair pulling, smoking, or spending too much money, or getting hooked on medications, drugs, or pills;

- wants to sort out problems like managing anger or coping with peer pressure;

- wants to build self-confidence or figure out ways to make more friends.

In short, therapy offers people support when they are going through difficult times.

Deciding to seek help for something you're going through can be really hard. It may be your idea to go to therapy or it might not. Sometimes parents or teachers bring up the idea first because they notice that someone they care about is dealing with a difficult situation, is losing weight, or seems unusually sad, worried, angry, or upset. Some people in this situation might welcome the idea or even feel relieved. Others might feel criticized or embarrassed and unsure if they'll benefit from talking to someone.

Sometimes people are told by teachers, parents, or the courts that they have to go see a therapist because they have been behaving in ways that are unacceptable, illegal, self-destructive, or dangerous. When therapy is someone else's idea, a person may at first feel like resisting the whole idea. But learning a bit more about what therapy involves and what to expect can help make it seem OK.

What Is Therapy?

Therapy isn't just for mental health. You've probably heard people discussing other types of medical therapy, such as physical therapy or chemotherapy. But the word "therapy" is most often used to mean psychotherapy (sometimes called "talk therapy")—in other words, psychological help to deal with stress or problems.

Psychotherapy is a process that's a lot like learning. Through therapy, people learn about themselves. They discover ways to overcome difficulties, develop inner strengths or skills, or make changes in themselves or their situations. Often, it feels good just to have a person to vent to, and other times it's useful to learn different techniques to help deal with stress.

> ## ✎ What's It Mean?
> A psychotherapist (therapist, for short) is a person who has been professionally trained to help people deal with stress or other problems. Psychiatrists, psychologists, social workers, counselors, and school psychologists are the titles of some of the licensed professionals who work as therapists. The letters following a therapist's name (for example, MD, PhD, PsyD, EdD, MA, LCSW, LPC) refer to the particular education and degree that therapist has received.

Some therapists specialize in working with a certain age group or on a particular type of problem. Other therapists treat a mix of ages and issues. Some work in hospitals, clinics, or counseling centers. Others work in schools or in psychotherapy offices, often called a "private practice" or "group practice."

What Do Therapists Do?

Most types of therapy include talking and listening, building trust, and receiving support and guidance. Sometimes therapists may recommend books for people to read or work through. They may also suggest keeping a journal. Some people prefer to express themselves using art or drawing. Others feel more comfortable just talking.

When a person talks to a therapist about which situations might be difficult for them or what stresses them out, this helps the therapist assess what is going on. The therapist and client then usually work together to set therapy goals and figure out what will help the person feel better or get back on track.

It might take a few meetings with a therapist before people really feel like they can share personal stuff. It's natural to feel that way. Trust is an essential ingredient in therapy—after all, therapy involves being open and honest about sensitive topics like feelings, ideas, relationships, problems, disappointments, and hopes. A therapist understands that people sometimes take a while to feel comfortable sharing personal information.

Most of the time, a person meets with a therapist one on one, which is known as individual therapy. Sometimes, though, a therapist might work with a family (called family therapy) or a group of people who all are dealing with similar issues (called group therapy or a support group). Family therapy gives family members a chance to talk together with a therapist about problems that involve them all. Group therapy and support groups help people give and receive support and learn from each other and their therapist by discussing the issues they have in common.

What Happens During Therapy?

If you see a therapist, he or she will talk with you about your feelings, thoughts, relationships, and important values. At the beginning, therapy sessions are focused on discussing what you'd like to work on and setting goals. Some of the goals people in therapy may set include things like:

- improving self-esteem and gaining confidence;
- figuring out how to make more friends;
- feeling less depressed or less anxious;
- improving grades at school;
- learning to manage anger and frustration;
- making healthier choices (for example, about relationships or eating) and ending self-defeating behaviors.

During the first visit, your therapist will probably ask you to talk a bit about yourself. Depending on your age, the therapist will also likely meet with a parent or caregiver and ask you to review information regarding confidentiality.

The first meeting can last longer than the usual "therapy hour" and is often called an "intake interview." This helps the therapist understand you better, and gives you a chance to see if you feel comfortable with the therapist. The therapist will probably ask about problems, concerns, and symptoms that you may be having, or the problems that parents or teachers are concerned about.

After one or two sessions, the therapist may talk to you about his or her understanding of what is going on with you, how therapy could help, and what the process will involve. Together, you and your therapist will decide on the goals for therapy and how frequently to meet. This may be once a week, every other week, or once a month.

With a better understanding of your situation, the therapist might teach you new skills or help you to think about a situation in a new way. For example, therapists can help people develop better relationship skills or coping skills, including ways to build confidence, express feelings, or manage anger.

Sticking to the schedule you agree on with your therapist and going to your appointments will ensure you have enough time with your therapist to work out your concerns. If your therapist suggests a schedule that you don't think you'll be able to keep, be up front about it so you can work out an alternative.

How Private Is It?

Therapists respect the privacy of their clients and they keep things they're told confidential. A therapist won't tell anyone else—including parents—about what a person discusses in his or her sessions unless that person gives permission. The only exception is if therapists believe their clients may harm themselves or others.

If the issue of privacy and confidentiality worries you, be sure to ask your therapist about it during your first meeting. It's important to feel comfortable with your therapist so you can talk openly about your situation.

Does It Mean I'm Crazy?

No. In fact, many people in your class have probably seen a therapist at some point—just like students often see tutors or coaches for extra help with schoolwork or sports. Getting help in dealing with emotions and stressful situations is as important to your overall health as getting help with a medical problem like asthma or diabetes.

There's nothing wrong with getting help with problems that are hard to solve alone. In fact, it's just the opposite. It takes a lot of courage and maturity to look for solutions to problems instead of ignoring or hiding them and allowing them to become worse. If you think that therapy could help you with a problem, ask an adult you trust—like a parent, school counselor, or doctor—to help you find a therapist.

A few adults still resist the idea of therapy because they don't fully understand it or have outdated ideas about it. A couple of generations ago, people didn't know as much about the mind or the mind-body connection as they do today, and people were left to struggle with their problems on their own. It used to be that therapy was only available to those with the most serious mental health problems, but that's no longer the case.

You don't have to hide the fact that you're going to a therapist, but you also don't have to tell anyone if you'd prefer not to. Some people find that talking to a few close friends about their therapy helps them to work out their problems and feel like they're not alone. Other people choose not to tell anyone, especially if they feel that others won't understand. Either way, it's a personal decision.

☞ Remember!!

Therapy is helpful to people of all ages and with problems that range from mild to much more serious. Some people still hold on to old beliefs about therapy, such as thinking that teens "will grow out of" their problems. If the adults in your family don't seem open to talking about therapy, mention your concerns to a school counselor, coach, or doctor.

What Can A Person Get Out Of Therapy?

What someone gets out of therapy depends on why that person is there. For example, some people go to therapy to solve a specific problem, others want to begin making better choices, and others want to start to heal from a loss or a difficult life situation.

Therapy can help people feel better, be stronger, and make good choices as well as discover more about themselves. Those who work with therapists might learn about motivations that lead them to behave in certain ways or about inner strengths they have. Maybe you'll learn new coping skills, develop more patience, or learn to like yourself better. Maybe you'll find new ways to handle problems that come up or new ways to handle yourself in tough situations.

People who work with therapists often find that they learn a lot about themselves and that therapy can help them grow and mature. Lots of people discover that the tools they learn in therapy when they're young make them feel stronger and better able to deal with whatever life throws at them even as adults. If you are curious about the therapy process, talk to a counselor or therapist to see if you could benefit.

Chapter 24

Medications For Treatment Of Mental Health Disorders

Medications are used to treat the symptoms of mental disorders such as schizophrenia, depression, bipolar disorder (sometimes called manic-depressive illness), anxiety disorders, and attention deficit-hyperactivity disorder (ADHD). Sometimes medications are used with other treatments such as psychotherapy.

Choosing the right medication, medication dose, and treatment plan should be based on a person's individual needs and medical situation, and under a doctor's care. Information about medications is frequently updated. Check the U.S. Food and Drug Administration (FDA) website for the latest information on warnings, patient medication guides, or newly approved medications (www.fda.gov).

Throughout this chapter you will see two names for medications—the generic name and in parenthesis, the trade name. An example is fluoxetine (Prozac).

About This Chapter: Text in this chapter is excerpted from "Mental Health Medications," National Institute of Mental Health (NIMH), 2009. The complete text of this document, including references and additional facts about side effects and related cautions, is available online at http://www.nimh.nih.gov/health/publications/mental-health-medications/introduction-mental-health-medications.shtml.

How are medications used to treat mental disorders?

Medications treat the symptoms of mental disorders. They cannot cure the disorder, but they make people feel better so they can function.

Medications work differently for different people. Some people get great results from medications and only need them for a short time. For example, a person with depression may feel much better after taking a medication for a few months, and may never need it again. People with disorders like schizophrenia or bipolar disorder, or people who have long-term or severe depression or anxiety may need to take medication for a much longer time.

Some people get side effects from medications and other people don't. Doses can be small or large, depending on the medication and the person. Factors that can affect how medic ations work in people include the following:

- Type of mental disorder, such as depression, anxiety, bipolar disorder, and schizophrenia

- Age, sex, and body size

- Physical illnesses

- Habits like smoking and drinking

- Liver and kidney function

- Genetics

- Other medications and herbal/vitamin supplements

- Diet

- Whether medications are taken as prescribed

> ### ✎ What's It Mean?
> ### What are psychiatric medications?
>
> Psychiatric medications treat mental disorders. Sometimes called psychotropic or psychotherapeutic medications, they have changed the lives of people with mental disorders for the better. Many people with mental disorders live fulfilling lives with the help of these medications. Without them, people with mental disorders might suffer serious and disabling symptoms.
>
> Source: National Institute of Mental Health, 2009.

What medications are used to treat depression?

Depression is commonly treated with antidepressant medications. Antidepressants work to balance some of the natural chemicals in our brains. These chemicals are called neurotransmitters, and they affect our mood and emotional responses. Antidepressants work on neurotransmitters such as serotonin, norepinephrine, and dopamine.

The most popular types of antidepressants are called selective serotonin reuptake inhibitors (SSRIs). These include the following:

- Fluoxetine (Prozac)
- Sertraline (Zoloft)
- Escitalopram (Lexapro)
- Citalopram (Celexa)
- Paroxetine (Paxil)

Other types of antidepressants are serotonin and norepinephrine reuptake inhibitors (SNRIs). SNRIs are similar to SSRIs and include venlafaxine (Effexor) and duloxetine (Cymbalta). Another antidepressant that is commonly used is bupropion (Wellbutrin). Bupropion, which works on the neurotransmitter dopamine, is unique in that it does not fit into any specific drug type.

SSRIs and SNRIs are popular because they do not cause as many side effects as older classes of antidepressants. Older antidepressant medications include tricyclics, tetracyclics, and monoamine oxidase inhibitors (MAOIs). For some people, tricyclics, tetracyclics, or MAOIs may be the best medications.

What are the side effects of antidepressants?

Antidepressants may cause mild side effects that usually do not last long. Any unusual reactions or side effects should be reported to a doctor immediately.

The most common side effects associated with SSRIs and SNRIs include these:

- Headache, which usually goes away within a few days
- Nausea (feeling sick to your stomach), which usually goes away within a few days
- Sleeplessness or drowsiness, which may happen during the first few weeks but then goes away. Sometimes the medication dose needs to be reduced or the time of day it is taken needs to be adjusted to help lessen these side effects.
- Agitation (feeling jittery)
- Sexual problems, which can affect both men and women and may include reduced sex drive, and problems having and enjoying sex

Tricyclic antidepressants can cause side effects, including the following:

- Dry mouth

- Constipation

- Bladder problems. It may be hard to empty the bladder, or the urine stream may not be as strong as usual. Older men with enlarged prostate conditions may be more affected.

- Sexual problems, which can affect both men and women and may include reduced sex drive, and problems having and enjoying sex

- Blurred vision, which usually goes away quickly

- Drowsiness. Usually, antidepressants that make you drowsy are taken at bedtime.

♣ It's A Fact!!

People taking monoamine oxidase inhibitors (MAO-Is) need to be careful about the foods they eat and the medicines they take. Foods and medicines that contain high levels of a chemical called tyramine are dangerous for people taking MAOIs. Tyramine is found in some cheeses, wines, and pickles. The chemical is also in some medications, including decongestants and over-the-counter cold medicine.

Mixing MAOIs and tyramine can cause a sharp increase in blood pressure, which can lead to stroke. People taking MAOIs should ask their doctors for a complete list of foods, medicines, and other substances to avoid. An MAOI skin patch has recently been developed and may help reduce some of these risks. A doctor can help a person figure out if a patch or a pill will work for him or her.

Source: National Institute of Mental Health, 2009.

How should antidepressants be taken?

People taking antidepressants need to follow their doctors' directions. The medication should be taken in the right dose for the right amount of time. It can take three or four weeks until the medicine takes effect. Some people take the medications for a short time, and some people take them for much longer periods. People with long-term or severe depression may need to take medication for a long time.

Once a person is taking antidepressants, it is important not to stop taking them without the help of a doctor. Sometimes people taking antidepressants feel better and stop taking the medication too soon, and the depression may return. When it is time to stop the medication, the doctor will help the person slowly and safely decrease the dose. It's important to give the body time to adjust to the change. People don't get addicted, or "hooked," on the medications, but stopping them abruptly can cause withdrawal symptoms.

If a medication does not work, it is helpful to be open to trying another one. A study funded by the National Institute of Mental Health (NIMH) found that if a person with difficult-to-treat depression did not get better with a first medication, chances of getting better increased when the person tried a new one or added a second medication to his or her treatment. The study was called STAR*D (Sequenced Treatment Alternatives to Relieve Depression).

Are herbal medicines used to treat depression?

The herbal medicine St. John's wort has been used for centuries in many folk and herbal remedies. Today in Europe, it is used widely to treat mild-to-moderate depression. In the United States, it is one of the top-selling botanical products.

The National Institutes of Health conducted a clinical trial to determine the effectiveness of treating adults who have major depression with St. John's wort. The study included 340 people diagnosed with major depression. One-third of the people took the herbal medicine, one-third took an SSRI, and one-third took a placebo, or "sugar pill." The people did not know what they were taking. The study found that St. John's wort was no more effective than the placebo in treating major depression. A study currently in progress is looking at the effectiveness of St. John's wort for treating mild or minor depression.

Other research has shown that St. John's wort can dangerously interact with other medications, including those used to control HIV. On February 10, 2000, the FDA issued a Public Health Advisory letter stating that the herb appears to interfere with certain medications used to treat heart disease, depression, seizures, certain cancers, and organ transplant rejection. Also, St. John's wort may interfere with oral contraceptives.

Because St. John's wort may not mix well with other medications, people should always talk with their doctors before taking it or any herbal supplement.

✤ It's A Fact!!
Depressed Adolescents Respond Best To Combination Treatment

A combination of psychotherapy and antidepressant medication appears to be the most effective treatment for adolescents with major depressive disorder—more than medication alone or psychotherapy alone, according to results from a major clinical trial funded by the National Institutes of Health's National Institute of Mental Health (NIMH). The study was published in the October 2007 issue of the *Archives of General Psychiatry*.

The long-term results of the Treatment for Adolescents with Depression Study (TADS) found that when adolescents received fluoxetine (Prozac) alone or in combination with cognitive behavioral therapy (CBT) over the course of 36 weeks, they recovered faster than those who were receiving CBT alone.

However, taking fluoxetine alone appeared to pose some safety concerns for the teens. During treatment, those taking fluoxetine alone had higher rates of suicidal thinking (15 percent) than those in combination treatment (eight percent) and those in CBT alone (six percent), particularly in the early stages of treatment. This suggests that while treatment with fluoxetine may speed recovery, adding CBT provides additional safeguards for those vulnerable to suicide, according to the researchers.

"Depression in teens is a serious illness that can and should be treated aggressively," said NIMH Director Thomas R. Insel, MD. "TADS provides compelling evidence for families and clinicians that the most effective way to treat depression in teens is with a two-pronged approach. It reassures us that antidepressant

Are antidepressants safe?

Antidepressants are safe and popular, but some studies have suggested that they may have unintentional effects, especially in young people. In 2004, the FDA looked at published and unpublished data on trials of antidepressants that involved nearly 4,400 children and adolescents. They found that 4 percent of those taking antidepressants thought about or tried suicide (although no suicides occurred), compared to two percent of those receiving placebos (sugar pill).

medication combined with psychotherapy is an effective and safe way to help teens recover from this disabling illness."

Results at 36 weeks of treatment were consistent with those found at 12 weeks in the 439-person study, when NIMH reported that combination treatment produced the greatest improvement in teenagers with major depression. At 18 weeks (results not previously reported), combination treatment still outpaced the other treatments with an 85 percent response rate, compared to 69 percent for fluoxetine alone and 65 percent for CBT alone. By 36 weeks, the response rate to combination treatment still remained the highest (86 percent), while response rates to fluoxetine and CBT essentially caught up, at 81 percent each.

"In the combination approach, the two treatments complemented each other," said John March, MD, MPH, of Duke University and lead author of the study. "The fluoxetine can help dissipate the physical symptoms of major depression relatively quickly, and CBT can help patients develop new skills to contend with difficult, negative emotions."

Because the trial sample included a mix of younger and older teens, both genders, substantial minority representation and variable socioeconomic status, the TADS results can be applied broadly to the adolescent population.

Source: From "Depressed Adolescents Respond Best to Combination Treatment," a Science Update from the National Institute of Mental Health, October 1, 2007.

In 2005, the FDA decided to adopt a "black box" warning label—the most serious type of warning—on all antidepressant medications. The warning says there is an increased risk of suicidal thinking or attempts in children and adolescents taking antidepressants. In 2007, the FDA proposed that makers of all antidepressant medications extend the warning to include young adults up through age 24.

The warning also says that patients of all ages taking antidepressants should be watched closely, especially during the first few weeks of treatment. Possible side effects to look for are depression that gets worse, suicidal thinking or behavior, or any unusual changes in behavior such as trouble sleeping, agitation, or withdrawal from normal social situations. Families and caregivers should report any changes to the doctor. To find the latest information visit the FDA website.

Results of a comprehensive review of pediatric trials conducted between 1988 and 2006 suggested that the benefits of antidepressant medications likely outweigh their risks to children and adolescents with major depression and anxiety disorders. The study was funded in part by NIMH.

Finally, the FDA has warned that combining the newer SSRI or SNRI antidepressants with one of the commonly-used "triptan" medications used to treat migraine headaches could cause a life-threatening illness called "serotonin syndrome." A person with serotonin syndrome may be agitated, have halluci-nations (see or hear things that are not real), have a high temperature, or have unusual blood pressure changes. Serotonin syndrome is usually associated with the older antidepressants called MAOIs, but it can happen with the newer antidepressants as well, if they are mixed with the wrong medications.

What medications are used to treat other types of mental illness?

Bipolar Disorder: Bipolar disorder, also called manic-depressive illness, is commonly treated with mood stabilizers. Sometimes, antipsychotics and antidepressants are used along with a mood stabilizer.

People with bipolar disorder usually try mood stabilizers first. In general, people continue treatment with mood stabilizers for years. Lithium is a very effective mood stabilizer. It was the first mood stabilizer approved by the FDA in the 1970s for treating both manic and depressive episodes.

✤ It's A Fact!!
Which groups have special needs
when taking psychiatric medications?

Psychiatric medications are taken by all types of people, but some groups, such as the following, have special needs:

• Children and adolescents

• Older adults

• Women who are pregnant or may become pregnant

• Children and adolescents

Most medications used to treat young people with mental illness are safe and effective. However, many medications have not been studied or approved for use with children. Researchers are not sure how these medications affect a child's growing body. Still, a doctor can give a young person a medication approved by the U.S. Food and Drug Administration (FDA)—an FDA-approved medication—on an "off-label" basis. This means that the doctor prescribes the medication to help the patient even though the medicine is not approved for the specific mental disorder or age.

For these reasons, it is important to watch young people who take these medications. Young people may have different reactions and side effects than adults. Also, some medications, including antidepressants and attention deficit-hyperactivity disorder (ADHD) medications, carry FDA warnings about potentially dangerous side effects for young people. See the sections on antidepressants and ADHD medications for more information about these warnings.

More research is needed on how these medications affect children and adolescents. NIMH has funded studies on this topic. For example, the National Institute of Mental Health (NIMH) funded the Preschoolers with ADHD Treatment Study (PATS), which involved 300 preschoolers (three to five years old) diagnosed with ADHD. The study found that low doses of the stimulant methylphenidate are safe and effective for preschoolers. However, children of this age are more sensitive to the side effects of the medication, including slower growth rates. Children taking methylphenidate should be watched closely.

In addition to medications, other treatments for young people with mental disorders should be considered. Psychotherapy, family therapy, educational courses, and behavior management techniques can help everyone involved cope with the disorder.

Source: National Institute of Mental Health, 2009.

Anticonvulsant medications also are used as mood stabilizers. They were originally developed to treat seizures, but they were found to help control moods as well. One anticonvulsant commonly used as a mood stabilizer is valproic acid, also called divalproex sodium (Depakote). For some people, it may work better than lithium. Other anticonvulsants used as mood stabilizers are carbamazepine (Tegretol), lamotrigine (Lamictal) and oxcarbazepine (Trileptal).

Anxiety Disorders: Anxiety disorders include obsessive compulsive disorder (OCD), post-traumatic stress disorder (PTSD), generalized anxiety disorder (GAD), panic disorder, and social phobia. Antidepressants, anti-anxiety medications, and beta-blockers are the most common medications used for anxiety disorders.

Antidepressants were developed to treat depression, but they also help people with anxiety disorders. SSRIs such as fluoxetine (Prozac), sertraline (Zoloft), escitalopram (Lexapro), paroxetine (Paxil), and citalopram (Celexa) are commonly prescribed for panic disorder, OCD, PTSD, and social phobia. The SNRI venlafaxine (Effexor) is commonly used to treat GAD. The antidepressant bupropion (Wellbutrin) is also sometimes used. When treating anxiety disorders, antidepressants generally are started at low doses and increased over time.

Some tricyclic antidepressants work well for anxiety. For example, imipramine (Tofranil) is prescribed for panic disorder and GAD. Clomipramine (Anafranil) is used to treat OCD. Tricyclics are also started at low doses and increased over time.

MAOIs are also used for anxiety disorders. Doctors sometimes prescribe phenelzine (Nardil), tranylcypromine (Parnate), and isocarboxazid (Marplan). People who take MAOIs must avoid certain food and medicines that can interact with their medicine and cause dangerous increases in blood pressure.

The anti-anxiety medications called benzodiazepines can start working more quickly than antidepressants. The ones used to treat anxiety disorders include the following:

- Clonazepam (Klonopin), which is used for social phobia and GAD

- Lorazepam (Ativan), which is used for panic disorder

- Alprazolam (Xanax), which is used for panic disorder and GAD

Buspirone (BuSpar) is an anti-anxiety medication used to treat GAD. Unlike benzodiazepines, however, it takes at least two weeks for buspirone to begin working.

Beta-blockers control some of the physical symptoms of anxiety, such as trembling and sweating. Propranolol (Inderal) is a beta-blocker usually used to treat heart conditions and high blood pressure. The medicine also helps people who have physical problems related to anxiety. For example, when a person with social phobia must face a stressful situation, such as giving a speech, or attending an important meeting, a doctor may prescribe a beta-blocker. Taking the medicine for a short period of time can help the person keep physical symptoms under control.

Schizophrenia: Antipsychotic medications are used to treat schizophrenia and schizophrenia-related disorders. Some of these medications have been available since the mid-1950s. They are also called conventional "typical" antipsychotics. Some of the more commonly used medications include the following:

- Chlorpromazine (Thorazine)
- Haloperidol (Haldol)
- Perphenazine (generic only)
- Fluphenazine (generic only)

In the 1990s, new antipsychotic medications were developed. These new medications are called second generation, or "atypical" antipsychotics. One of these medications was clozapine (Clozaril). It is a very effective medication that treats psychotic symptoms, hallucinations, and breaks with reality, such as when a person believes he or she is the president. But clozapine can sometimes cause a serious problem called agranulocytosis, which is a loss of the white blood cells that help a person fight infection. Therefore, people who take clozapine must get their white blood cell counts checked every week or two. This problem and the cost of blood tests make treatment with clozapine difficult for many people. Still, clozapine is potentially helpful for people who do not respond to other antipsychotic medications.

Other atypical antipsychotics were developed. All of them are effective, and none cause agranulocytosis. These include the following:

- Risperidone (Risperdal)
- Olanzapine (Zyprexa)
- Quetiapine (Seroquel)
- Ziprasidone (Geodon)
- Aripiprazole (Abilify)
- Paliperidone (Invega)

Chapter 25

Dealing With Addiction

Jason's life is beginning to unravel. His grades have slipped, he's moody, he doesn't talk to his friends, and he has stopped showing up for practice. Jason's friends know he has been experimenting with drugs, and now they're worried he has become addicted.

Defining an addiction is tricky, and knowing how to handle one is even harder.

What Are Substance Abuse And Addiction?

The difference between substance abuse and addiction is very slight. Substance abuse means using an illegal substance or using a legal substance in the wrong way. Addiction begins as abuse, or using a substance like marijuana or cocaine. You can abuse a drug (or alcohol) without having an addiction. For example, just because Sara smoked weed a few times doesn't mean that she has an addiction, but it does mean that she's abusing a drug—and that could lead to an addiction.

People can get addicted to all sorts of substances. When we think of addiction, we usually think of alcohol or illegal drugs. But people become addicted to medications, cigarettes, even glue. And some substances are more addictive than others: Drugs like crack or heroin are so addictive that they might only be used once or twice before the user loses control.

Addiction means a person has no control over whether he or she uses a drug or drinks. Someone who's addicted to cocaine has grown so used to the drug that he or she has to have it. Addiction can be physical, psychological, or both.

Physical Addiction

Being physically addicted means a person's body actually becomes dependent on a particular substance (even smoking is physically addictive). It also means building tolerance to that substance, so that a person needs a larger dose than ever before to get the same effects. Someone who is physically addicted and stops using a substance like drugs, alcohol, or cigarettes may experience withdrawal symptoms. Common symptoms of withdrawal are diarrhea, shaking, and generally feeling awful.

Psychological Addiction

Psychological addiction happens when the cravings for a drug are psychological or emotional. People who are psychologically addicted feel overcome by the desire to have a drug. They may lie or steal to get it.

A person crosses the line between abuse and addiction when he or she is no longer trying the drug to have fun or get high, but has come to depend on it. His or her whole life centers around the need for the drug. An addicted person—whether it's a physical or psychological addiction or both—no longer feels like there is a choice in taking a substance.

Signs Of Addiction

The most obvious sign of an addiction is the need to have a particular drug or substance. However, many other signs can suggest a possible addiction, such as changes in mood or weight loss or gain. (These also are signs of other conditions, too, though, such as depression or eating disorders.)

Signs that you or someone you know may have a drug or alcohol addiction include:

♣ It's A Fact!!
Introducing... Your Brain

The brain is the command center of your body. It controls just about everything you do, even when you are sleeping.

Weighing about three pounds, the brain is made up of many parts that all work together as a team. Each of these different parts has a specific and important job to do.

When drugs enter the brain, they can interrupt the work and actually change how the brain performs its jobs. These changes are what lead to compulsive drug use, the hallmark of addiction.

Drugs of abuse affect three primary areas of the brain:

The Brain Stem: This area of the brain is in charge of all of the functions our body needs to stay alive—breathing, circulating blood, and digesting food. It also links the brain with the spinal cord, which runs down the back and is responsible for moving muscles and limbs as well as letting the brain know what's happening to the body.

The Limbic System: This system links together a bunch of brain structures that control our emotional responses, such as feeling pleasure when we eat chocolate. The good feelings motivate us to repeat the behavior, which is good because eating is critical to our lives.

The Cerebral Cortex: This part of the brain is the mushroom-like outer part of the brain (the gray matter). In humans, it is so big that it makes up about three-fourths of the entire brain. It's divided into four areas, called lobes, which control specific functions. Some areas process information from our senses, enabling us to see, feel, hear, and taste. The front part of the cortex, known as the frontal cortex or forebrain, is the thinking center. It powers our ability to think, plan, solve problems, and make decisions.

Source: Excerpted from "Brain and Addiction," National Institute on Drug Abuse, November 2007.

Psychological Signals

- Use of drugs or alcohol as a way to forget problems or to relax
- Withdrawal or keeping secrets from family and friends
- Loss of interest in activities that used to be important
- Problems with schoolwork, such as slipping grades or absences
- Changes in friendships, such as hanging out only with friends who use drugs
- Spending a lot of time figuring out how to get drugs
- Stealing or selling belongings to be able to afford drugs
- Failed attempts to stop taking drugs or drinking
- Anxiety, anger, or depression
- Mood swings

Physical Signals

- Changes in sleeping habits
- Feeling shaky or sick when trying to stop
- Needing to take more of the substance to get the same effect
- Changes in eating habits, including weight loss or gain

Getting Help

If you think you're addicted to drugs or alcohol, recognizing that you have a problem is the first step in getting help.

A lot of people think they can kick the problem on their own, but that doesn't work for most people. Find someone you trust to talk to. It may help to talk to a friend or someone your own age at first, but a supportive and understanding adult is your best option for getting help. If you can't talk to your parents, you might want to approach a school counselor, relative, doctor, favorite teacher, or religious leader.

Unfortunately, overcoming addiction is not easy. Quitting drugs or drinking is probably going to be one of the hardest things you've ever done. It's not a sign of weakness if you need professional help from a trained drug counselor or therapist. Most people who try to kick a drug or alcohol problem need professional assistance or a treatment program to do so.

✣ It's A Fact!!
How does the brain communicate?

The brain is a complex communications network consisting of billions of neurons, or nerve cells. Networks of neurons pass messages back and forth within the brain, the spinal column, and the peripheral nervous system. These nerve networks control everything we feel, think, and do.

- **Neurons:** Your brain contains about 100 billion neurons—nerve cells that work nonstop to send and receive messages. Within a neuron, messages travel from the cell body down the axon to the axon terminal in the form of electrical impulses. From there, the message is sent to other neurons with the help of neurotransmitters.

- **Neurotransmitters—The Brain's Chemical Messengers:** To make messages jump from one neuron to another, the neuron creates chemical messengers, called neurotransmitters. The axon terminal releases neurotransmitters that travel across the space (called the synapse) to nearby neurons. Then the transmitter binds to receptors on the nearby neuron.

- **Receptors—The Brain's Chemical Receivers:** As the neurotransmitter approaches the nearby neuron, it attaches to a special site on the cell called a receptor. A neurotransmitter and its receptor operate like a key and lock, in that an exquisitely specific mechanism makes sure that each receptor will forward the appropriate message only after interacting with the right kind of neurotransmitter.

- **Transporters—The Brain's Chemical Recyclers:** Once neurotransmitters do their job, they are pulled back into their original neuron by transporters. This recycling process shuts off the signal between the neurons.

To send a message, a brain cell releases a chemical (neurotransmitter) into the space separating two cells, called the synapse. The neurotransmitter crosses the synapse and attaches to proteins (receptors) on the receiving brain cell. This causes changes in the receiving brain cell, and the message is delivered.

Source: Excerpted from "Brain and Addiction," National Institute on Drug Abuse, November 2007.

Tips For Recovery

Once you start a treatment program, try these tips to make the road to recovery less bumpy:

Tell your friends about your decision to stop using drugs: Your true friends will respect your decision. This might mean that you need to find a new group of friends who will be 100 percent supportive. Unless everyone decides to kick their drug habit at once, you probably won't be able to hang out with the friends you did drugs with before.

Ask your friends or family to be available when you need them. You may need to call someone in the middle of the night just to talk. If you're going through a tough time, don't try to handle things on your own—accept the help your family and friends offer.

Accept invitations only to events that you know won't involve drugs or alcohol. Going to the movies is probably safe, but you may want to skip a Friday night party until you're feeling more secure. Plan activities that don't involve drugs. Go to the movies, try bowling, or take an art class with a friend.

Have a plan about what you'll do if you find yourself in a place with drugs or alcohol: The temptation will be there sometimes, but if you know how you're going to handle it, you'll be OK. Establish a plan with your parents or siblings so that if you call home using a code, they'll know that your call is a signal you need a ride out of there.

Remind yourself that having an addiction doesn't make you bad or weak. If you fall back into old patterns (backslide) a bit, talk to an adult as soon as possible. There's nothing to be ashamed about, but it's important to get help soon so that all of the hard work you put into your recovery is not lost.

If you're worried about a friend who has an addiction, use these tips to help him or her, too: For example, let your friend know that you are available to talk or offer your support. If you notice a friend backsliding, talk about it openly and ask what you can do to help. If your friend is going back to drugs or drinking and won't accept your help, don't be afraid to talk to a nonthreatening, understanding adult, like your parent or school counselor. It may seem like you're ratting your friend out, but it's the best support you can offer.

Above all, offer a friend who's battling an addiction lots of encouragement and praise. It may seem corny, but hearing that you care is just the kind of motivation your friend needs.

♣ It's A Fact!!
What do drugs do to the brain?

Drugs are chemicals. They work in the brain by tapping into its communication system and interfering with the way nerve cells normally send, receive, and process information. Different drugs—because of their chemical structures—work differently. In fact, some drugs can change the brain in ways that last long after the person has stopped taking drugs, maybe even permanently. This is more likely when a drug is taken repeatedly.

Some drugs, such as marijuana and heroin, activate neurons because their chemical structure mimics that of a natural neurotransmitter. In fact, these drugs can "fool" receptors, can lock onto them, and can activate the nerve cells. The problem is, they don't work the same way as a natural neurotransmitter, so the neurons wind up sending abnormal messages through the brain.

Other drugs, such as amphetamine, cause nerve cells to release excessive amounts of natural neurotransmitters or prevent the normal recycling of these brain chemicals (cocaine and amphetamine). This leads to an exaggerated message in the brain, ultimately wreaking havoc on the communication channels. The difference in effect is like the difference between someone whispering in your ear versus someone shouting in a microphone.

All drugs of abuse, nicotine, cocaine, marijuana, and others, affect the brain's "reward" circuit, which is part of the limbic system. Normally, the reward circuit responds to pleasurable experiences by releasing the neurotransmitter dopamine, which creates feelings of pleasure, and tells the brain that this is something important—pay attention and remember it. Drugs hijack this system, causing unusually large amounts of dopamine to flood the system. Sometimes, this lasts for a long time compared to what happens when a natural reward stimulates dopamine. This flood of dopamine is what causes the "high" or euphoria associated with drug abuse.

Source: Excerpted from "Brain and Addiction," National Institute on Drug Abuse, November 2007.

Staying Clean

Recovering from a drug or alcohol addiction doesn't end with a six-week treatment program. It's a lifelong process. Many people find that joining a support group can help them stay clean. There are support groups specifically for teens and younger people. You'll meet people who have gone through the same experiences you have, and you'll be able to participate in real-life discussions about drugs that you won't hear in your school's health class.

Many people find that helping others is also the best way to help themselves. Your understanding of how difficult the recovery process can be will help you to support others—both teens and adults—who are battling an addiction.

If you do have a relapse, recognizing the problem as soon as possible is critical. Get help right away so that you don't undo all the hard work you put into your initial recovery. And, if you do have a relapse, don't ever be afraid to ask for help.

Chapter 26

Recovering From A Suicide Attempt

This information was developed to help you as you begin to work through the challenges that led you to attempt to take your life. It offers information about moving ahead after your treatment in the emergency department and provides resources for more information about suicide and mental illnesses.

Today

Today may feel like the hardest day of your life. You have seriously thought about or perhaps attempted to end your life. You may be exhausted. A common experience after surviving a suicide attempt is extreme fatigue. You may be angry. You may be embarrassed or ashamed. The attempt itself, the reactions of other people, transportation to and treatment in an emergency department or other health care facility—all these can be overwhelming to you right now. But recovery is likely, and all the feelings you are experiencing right now can get better.

After The Emergency Department

After you have been treated for a suicide attempt in an emergency department and the doctors believe you are medically stabilized, you will either be discharged (released) or you will be hospitalized.

About This Chapter: Information in this chapter is excerpted from "After an Attempt: A Guide for Taking Care of Yourself after Your Treatment in the Emergency Department," Substance Abuse and Mental Health Services Administration (www.samhsa.gov), 2006.

If you are discharged after your suicide attempt, the staff in the emergency department should provide you with a plan for follow-up care. The exact steps for follow-up care will vary with each person, but your plan should include these elements:

- A scheduled appointment in the near future with a mental health provider (such as a psychiatrist or other licensed therapist). Make sure that the name and contact information for the provider is given to you before you leave the hospital and that your appointment will occur as soon as possible.

- Information on any treatments that you received in the emergency department, such as medications, and what, if anything, you will need to do about those treatments after you leave.

- Referrals to local and national resources and crisis lines for information and support.

Once you have a plan for follow-up care that you understand and are comfortable with, you and, if appropriate, a family member should work closely with a therapist to ensure that your plan is meaningful and effective. If the emergency department staff feel that you need more immediate care or longer-term care than the emergency department can provide, you will be referred for inpatient hospitalization. If hospitalization is necessary, you and your family, if appropriate, can begin to work with the hospital to develop a plan for the next steps in your care. Hospital staff (usually a social worker) should help you with this process.

What If You Don't Want To Go To The Hospital?

People generally have the right to consent to or refuse treatment. However, if the emergency physician believes you are a danger to yourself or someone else, he or she must consider having you hospitalized involuntarily for a limited period of time.

Laws about commitment vary by state. If you have questions about your rights as a patient, you should contact your local Protection and Advocacy organization. These are legal centers that are funded to protect the rights of persons with mental health needs. You can either go to their national website at www.ndrn.org or call the office at 202-408-9514 to inquire about the Protection and Advocacy center in your state.

Next Steps: Moving Ahead And Coping With Future Thoughts Of Suicide

Recovery from the negative thoughts and feelings that made you want to end your life is possible. You may get to a place where you never have thoughts of suicide again and you can lead a happy, satisfying life. You also may learn to live with these thoughts in a way that keeps you safe.

After you leave the hospital there are several things you can do to help in your recovery. It may feel hard and overwhelming right now, but over the next few days, following these tips can help turn things around.

Create a safety plan: You and your doctor, or other licensed therapist, should work together to develop a safety plan to help reduce the risk of a future suicide attempt. When creating a safety plan, be honest with yourself and your doctor to ensure that the plan meets your needs and that you feel comfortable with it. Although everyone's safety plan is different, the following are some common things that may be in your plan:

- Signs that may indicate a return of suicidal thoughts or feelings and what to do about them

- When to seek additional treatment

- Contact information for your doctor, therapist, or a trusted friend or family member

Keep a written copy of your safety plan nearby so you can refer to it as needed.

Build a support system: A support system is a key part of recovering from a suicide attempt and preventing another one. It is important that you have at least one person in your life who can be your "ally." This must be a person you trust and can be honest with—especially if you start to have thoughts of ending your life again.

Family members or a close friend can serve this important purpose. A member of the clergy, mentor, or colleague also could be helpful to you at this time. Having more than one ally can be a great asset, as well. Keeping your ally informed about your thoughts, feelings, and wishes can help in your recovery and may help prevent another suicide attempt. You will have to be honest with yourself and with your ally to make this work. Even when you are feeling alone, always remember that there are people in your life who care about you a great deal and are willing to help.

Learn to live again: When you are recovering, the world can look like a pretty bleak place. It may take a little while before your life starts to feel comfortable again. One thing you can do to help is to get back into a routine. Eat at regular

---

✔ Quick Tip

- Remove the means for hurting yourself from your environment. Work with your ally to remove methods of self-harm. It is better not to have these things around while you are recovering. If you use medication, keep only a few days' supply on hand and ask someone else to hold onto the rest. For other means of self-harm, place them in someone else's hands for a while. You can always take back these items when things feel more settled.

- Identify what sets off or starts these thoughts for you. It may be an anniversary of painful event, for instance, or seeing a knife in the kitchen. Plan to minimize the effect of these triggers on your life. Sometimes you can avoid them or train yourself to respond differently, or you can involve your allies ahead of time to help you face a difficult situation. Remember that life events do not cause a suicide, but they can increase the risk of an attempt.

- Learn about mental illness. Someone who has had or is living with suicidal thoughts may be suffering from a mental illness such as bipolar disorder, schizophrenia, or major depression.

- Learn about crisis hotlines. Hotlines provide you with a trained person to talk to when you are having suicidal thoughts. This person will listen to you and help you choose another path. The person you talk with may work with you on your safety plan, so have that plan close by when you make the call. If you do not have a safety plan in place, the crisis staff will help you create one.

- Participate in a mutual peer-support group. There are many types of support groups, and you may wish to participate in one in your area. Learning from others and sharing your experience can make a big difference in the way you think about your life. It also may help save the life of someone else.

times, exercise regularly, and go to sleep and get up at the same time each day. Try to join in your usual activities a little at a time, and add in more when you feel comfortable If you continue to have thoughts of suicide, reach out for help immediately and contact your ally, a doctor, or a crisis hotline (see the back pages of this brochure for listings). Remember, the emergency department is open 24 hours a day, 365 days a year to help you if you have thoughts of suicide or if your medical team is unavailable to provide you with the needed care.

Listen closely, and carefully consider the support and advice you receive. It is important to be honest with yourself, your doctor, or others about your feelings so that you get the best possible care.

Sometimes being under pressure and having thoughts of suicide can make it difficult for you to make the best decisions, and at those times, other people may have a more realistic view of your situation than you do. Your ally can help you work through these confusing and isolating thoughts and feelings and help keep you safe.

Everyone's recovery is different: Some people have persistent thoughts of suicide. For others, such thoughts may accompany certain moods or circumstances. Here are some steps you can take to prevent negative and destructive thoughts in the future and to keep you safe. You also may want to consider adding some of these steps to your safety plan.

Get involved in life: Finding a hobby or enjoying a favorite pastime—such as listening to music, watching your favorite movie, or collecting things—is a great way to help you cope when things get tough. Hobbies or activities that involve interacting with others are an especially good idea. Whatever your interests may be, make sure you have access to the things you enjoy. That way, if your negative thoughts come back, you can turn to something that brings you comfort and enjoyment.

☞ Remember!!
There are reasons to live and make things better. You can survive, and even thrive, despite the way you feel at times. Recovery is likely.

Chapter 27

Helping Someone Else Recovering From A Suicide Attempt

Suicidal thoughts and actions generate conflicting feelings in family members who love the person who wishes to take his or her own life. That is why this information was developed for you. It will give you some important points on how to take care of yourself and your family member following a suicide attempt and it will provide resources to help you move forward.

What Happens In The Emergency Department

Goal

The goal of an emergency department visit is to get the best outcome for the person at a time of crisis—resolving the crisis, stabilizing the patient medically and emotionally, and making recommendations and referrals for follow-up care or treatment. There are several steps in the process, and they all take time.

When someone is admitted to an emergency department for a suicide attempt, a doctor will evaluate the person's physical and mental health.

About This Chapter: Text in this chapter is from "After an Attempt: A Guide For Taking Care of Your Family Member after Treatment in the Emergency Department," Substance Abuse and Mental Health Services Administration (www.samhsa.gov), 2006.

Emergency department staff should look for underlying physical problems that may have contributed to the suicidal behavior, such as side effects from medications, untreated medical conditions, or the presence of street drugs that can cause emotional distress. While emergency department staff prefer to assess people who are sober, they should not dismiss things people say or do when intoxicated, especially comments about how they might harm themselves or others.

Assessment

After emergency department staff evaluate your family member's physical health, a mental health assessment should be performed, and the physician doing the exam should put your relative's suicidal behavior into context. The assessment will generally focus on three areas:

1. What psychiatric or medical conditions are present? Are they being or have they been treated? Are the suicidal thoughts and behavior a result of a recent change, or are they a longstanding condition?

2. What did the person do to harm himself or herself? Have there been previous attempts? Why did the person act, and why now? What current stressors, including financial or relationship losses, may have contributed to this decision? Does the person regret surviving the suicide attempt? Is the person angry with someone? Is the person trying to reunite with someone who has died? What is the person's perspective on death?

🖙 Remember!!

Inform the emergency department personnel if your relative has:

- Access to a gun, lethal doses of medications, or other means of suicide;

- Stopped taking prescribed medicines;

- Stopped seeing a mental health provider or physician;

- Written a suicide note or will;

- Given possessions away;

- Been in or is currently in an abusive relationship;

- An upcoming anniversary of a loss;

- Started abusing alcohol or drugs;

- Recovered well from a previous suicidal crisis following a certain type of intervention.

3. What support systems are there? Who is providing treatment? What treatment programs are a good match for the person? What does the individual and the family feel comfortable with? Finally, a doctor may assess in more detail the actual suicide attempt that brought your relative into the emergency department. Information that the treatment team should look for includes the presence of a suicide note, the seriousness of the attempt, or a history of previous suicide attempts.

What The Emergency Department Needs To Know: How You Can Help

Confidentiality And Information Sharing

Family members are a source of history and are often key to the discharge plan. Provide as much information as possible to the emergency department staff. Even if confidentiality laws prevent the medical staff from giving you information about your relative, you can always give them information. Find out who is doing the evaluation and talk with that person. You can offer information that may influence the decisions made for your relative.

If you ever again have to accompany your relative to the emergency department after an attempt, remember to bring all medications, suspected causes of overdose, and any names and phone numbers of providers who may have information. Emergency department personnel should try to contact the medical professionals who know the situation best before making decisions.

Other important information about your relative's history to share with the emergency department staff include:

- A family history of actual suicide—mental health professionals are taught to pay attention to this because there is an increased risk in families with a history of suicide.

- Details about your relative's treatment team—a recent change in medication, the therapist is on vacation, etc. This information is relevant for emergency department staff because if they do not feel hospitalization is best, they need to discharge your family member to a professional's care.

- If the person has an advance directive, review this with the emergency department treatment team. If you have a guardianship, let them know that as well. You may want to get permission from the staff and your relative to sit in on your relative's evaluation in the emergency department to listen and add information as needed. Your role is to balance the emergency department staff's training and the interview of the patient with your perspective. The best emergency department decisions are made with all the relevant information.

✎ **What's It Mean?**

Advance directives are legal documents that allow someone to give directions for future medical care or designate another person to make medical decisions if one is unable to competently make such decisions.

Next Steps After The Emergency Department

After your relative's physical and mental health are thoroughly examined, the emergency department personnel will decide if your relative needs to be hospitalized—either voluntarily or by a commitment. If hospitalization is necessary, you can begin to work with the receiving hospital to offer information and support and to develop a plan for the next steps in your relative's care. If involuntary hospitalization is necessary, the hospital staff should explain this legal procedure to your relative and you so that you both have a clear understanding of what will take place over the next three to ten days, while a court decides on the next steps for treatment.

If your relative has a hearing impairment or does not speak English, he or she may have to wait for someone who knows American Sign Language or an interpreter. It is generally not a good idea to use a family member to interpret in a medical situation. If the emergency department's treatment team, the patient, and you do not feel hospitalization is necessary, then you should all be a part of developing a follow-up treatment plan.

Questions Family And Friends Should Ask About The Follow-up Treatment Plan

Ask your family member these questions. It is important to be honest and direct with your questions and concerns.

• Do you feel safe to leave the hospital, and are you comfortable with the discharge plan?

- How is your relationship with your doctor, and when is your next appointment?

- What has changed since your suicidal feelings or actions began?

- What else can I/we do to help you after you leave the emergency department?

- Will you agree to talk with me/us if your suicidal feelings return? If not, is there someone else you can talk to?

Ask the treatment team these questions. This includes the doctor, therapist, nurse, social worker, etc.:

- Do you believe professionally that my family member is ready to leave the hospital?

- Why did you make the decision(s) that you did about my family member's care or treatment?

- Is there a follow-up appointment scheduled? Can it be moved to an earlier date?

- What is my role as a family member in the safety plan?

- What should we look for and when should we seek more help, such as returning to the emergency department or contacting other local resources and providers?

What You Need To Know

Make safety a priority for your relative recovering from a suicide attempt. Research has shown that a person who has attempted to end his or her life has a much higher risk of later dying by suicide. Safety is ultimately an individual's responsibility, but often a person who feels suicidal has a difficult time making good choices. As a family member, you can help your loved one make a better choice while reducing the risk.

☞ Remember!!
It is critical for the patient to schedule a follow-up appointment as soon as possible after discharge from the emergency department.

Reduce The Risk At Home

To help reduce the risk of self-harm or suicide at home, here are some things to consider:

• Guns are high risk and the leading means of death for suicidal people—they should be taken out of the home and secured.

• Overdoses are common and can be lethal—if it is necessary to keep pain relievers such as aspirin, Advil, and Tylenol in the home, only keep small quantities or consider keeping medications in a locked container. Remove unused or expired medicine from the home.

• Alcohol use or abuse can decrease inhibitions and cause people to act more freely on their feelings. As with pain relievers, keep only small quantities of alcohol in the home, if none at all.

Create A Safety Plan

Following a suicide attempt, a safety plan should be created to help prevent another attempt. The plan should be a joint effort between your relative and his or her doctor, therapist, or the emergency department staff, and you. As a family member, you should know your relative's safety plan and understand your role in it, including the following:

• Knowing your family member's "triggers," such as an anniversary of a loss, alcohol, or stress from relationships.

• Building supports for your family member with mental health professionals, family, friends, and community resources.

• Working with your family member's strengths to promote his or her safety.

• Promoting communication and honesty in your relationship with your family member.

Remember that safety cannot be guaranteed by anyone—the goal is to reduce the risks and build supports for everyone in the family. However, it is important for you to believe that the safety plan can help keep your relative safe. If you do not feel that it can, let the emergency department staff know before you leave.

Maintain Hope And Self-Care

Families commonly provide a safety net and a vision of hope for their suicidal relative, and that can be emotionally exhausting. Never try to handle this situation alone—get support from friends, relatives, and organizations such as the National Alliance on Mental Illness, and get professional input whenever possible. You do not have to travel this road alone.

Moving Forward

Emergency department care is by nature short-term and crisis oriented, but some longer-term interventions have been shown to help reduce suicidal behavior and thoughts. You and your relative can talk to the doctor about various treatments for mental illnesses that may help to reduce the risk of suicide for people diagnosed with illnesses such as schizophrenia, bipolar disorder, or depression. Often, these illnesses require multiple types of interventions, and your relative may benefit from a second opinion from a specialist.

If your relative abuses alcohol or other drugs, it is also important to seek help for this problem along with the suicidal behavior. Seek out a substance abuse specialist.

Ultimately, please reach out for help in supporting your family member and yourself through this crisis. See the list below of hotlines, information, and support organizations to help you and your family member move forward with your lives.

Remember that the emergency department is open 24 hours a day, 365 days a year to treat your family member, if the problem continues and if your family member's medical team is unavailable to provide the needed care.

Part Four

When Someone You Know
Dies From Suicide

Chapter 28

Surviving Suicide Loss

Coming to terms with the death of a loved one is one of life's most challenging journeys. When the death is from suicide, family members and friends can experience an even more complex kind of grief. While trying to cope with the pain of their sudden loss, they are overwhelmed by feelings of blame, anger and incomprehension. Adding to their burden is the stigma that still surrounds suicide.

Survivors of suicide and their friends can help each other and themselves by gaining an understanding of grief after suicide. For survivors, it helps to know that the intensity of their feelings is normal. Friends can learn how to support the bereaved.

A Different Grief

Survivors of suicide—the family and friends of a person who completes suicide—feel the emotions that death always brings. Adding to their suffering is the shock of a sudden, often unexpected death. As well, they may feel isolated and judged by society, friends, and colleagues.

Some people compare the emotional stress to being trapped on an endless roller coaster.

About This Chapter: Text in this chapter is from "Grief After Suicide," © 2009 Canadian Mental Health Association (www.cmha.ca). Reprinted with permission.

Survivors may feel:

- guilt, anger, blame, shame, confusion, relief, despair, betrayal, abandonment;

- disconnected from their loved one because he or she chose to die;

- consumed by a need to find the meaning and reasons for the suicide;

- an exaggerated sense of responsibility for the death;

- the suicide was malicious, or a way for the deceased to get back at them.

Stigma Affects Mourning

Suicide is a difficult topic for many people. Cultural and religious taboos can lead to judgmental or condemning attitudes. Some people prefer to avoid even discussing suicide and their lack of knowledge about it makes them fearful. Attitudes like these can isolate and further stress survivors.

Stigma leads survivors to feel abandoned by their social network. They describe:

- being avoided by friends or acquaintances;

- feeling judged;

- people behaving as if the death had not occurred.

Some survivors perceive stigma that is not really there. They may anticipate difficult questions and disapproval, and withdraw in order to protect themselves.

✤ It's A Fact!!

A survivor of suicide is a family member or friend of a person who died by suicide.

Some Facts

Survivors of suicide represent "the largest mental health casualties related to suicide" (Edwin Shneidman, PhD, American Association of Suicidology, Founding President).

There are currently over 32,000 suicides annually in the USA. It is estimated that for every suicide there are at least six survivors. Some suicidologists believe this to be a very conservative estimate.

Based on this estimate, approximately five million American became survivors of suicide in the last 25 years.

Source: Excerpted from "Survivors of Suicide Fact Sheet," © 2007 American Association of Suicidology (www.suicidology.org). Reprinted with permission.

Whether it is real or perceived, stigma can affect a survivor's journey to acceptance.

What Survivors Should Know

First, know that you are not alone. Approximately one out of four people know someone who died by suicide. It can also help to know that suicide was the decision of the person who died. It is estimated that the majority of suicides are the result of untreated depression or other mental illness.

Survivors Are At Risk

Survivors of suicide are at high risk of completing suicide themselves. The experience suddenly makes the idea of suicide very real, and it is not uncommon for survivors to experience suicidal thoughts. Another factor is that suicide-related illnesses like depression run in families.

Because of this increased risk for suicide, survivors should not be isolated, but rather supported and encouraged to talk about all their feelings—even the most difficult ones.

✤ It's A Fact!!
About Suicidal Grief

The loss of a loved one by suicide is often shocking, painful and unexpected. The grief that ensues can be intense, complex, and long term. Grief work is an extremely individual and unique process; each person will experience it in their own way and at their own pace.

Grief does not follow a linear path. Furthermore, grief doesn't always move in a forward direction.

There is no time frame for grief. Survivors should not expect that their lives will return to their prior state. Survivors aim to adjust to life without their loved one.

Source: Excerpted from "Survivors of Suicide Fact Sheet," © 2007 American Association of Suicidology (www .suicidology.org). Reprinted with permission.

Survivor Coping Strategies

No two people ever experience grief in the same way, or with the same intensity, but there are strategies that can help you cope with your loss.

- Acknowledge that the death is a suicide.

- Recognize your feelings and loss.

- Talk openly with your family so that everyone's grief is acknowledged and can be expressed.

- Reach out to your friends and guide them if they don't know what to say or do.

- Find support groups where you can share your stories, memories and methods of coping.

- Be aware that anniversaries (e.g., birthdays) can be especially difficult and consider whether to continue old traditions or begin new ones.

- Develop rituals to honor your loved one's life.

How Can I Help My Friend?

Showing a willingness to listen is probably the most important thing you can do for a friend who is a survivor of suicide. It may be distressing at first, but you're not expected to provide answers. Instead, you can be a comforting, safe place for someone who desperately needs to talk.

☞ **Remember!!**

Common emotions experienced in grief are:

- Shock
- Denial
- Pain
- Guilt
- Anger
- Shame
- Despair
- Disbelief
- Hopelessness
- Stress
- Sadness
- Numbness
- Rejection
- Loneliness
- Abandonment
- Confusion
- Self-blame
- Anxiety
- Helplessness
- Depression

These feelings are normal reactions and the expression of them is a natural part or grieving. At first, and periodically during the following days/months of grieving, survivors may feel overwhelmed by their emotions. It is important to take things one day at a time.

Source: Excerpted from "Survivors of Suicide Fact Sheet," © 2007 American Association of Suicidology (www.suicidology.org). Reprinted with permission.

❖ It's A Fact!!

Crying is the expression of sadness; it is therefore a natural reaction after the loss of a loved one.

Survivors often struggle with the reasons why the suicide occurred and whether they could have done something to prevent the suicide or help their loved one. Feelings of guilt typically ensue if the survivor believes their loved one's suicide could have been prevented.

At times, especially if the loved one had a mental disorder, the survivor may experience relief.

There is a stigma attached to suicide, partly due to the misunderstanding surrounding it. As such, family members and friends of the survivor may not know what to say or how and when to provide assistance. They may rely on the survivor's initiative to talk about the loved one or to ask for help.

Shame or embarrassment might prevent the survivor from reaching out for help. Stigma, ignorance and uncertainty might prevent others from giving the necessary support and understanding. Ongoing support remains important to maintain family and friendship relations during the grieving process.

Survivors sometimes feel that others are blaming them for the suicide. Survivors may feel the need to deny what happened or hide their feelings. This will most likely exacerbate and complicate the grieving process.

When the time is right, survivors will begin to enjoy life again. Healing does occur.

Many survivors find that the best help comes from attending a support group for survivors of suicide where they can openly share their own story and their feelings with fellow survivors without pressure or fear of judgment and shame. Support groups can be a helpful source of guidance and understanding as well as a support in the healing process.

Source: Excerpted from "Survivors of Suicide Fact Sheet," © 2007 American Association of Suicidology (www.suicidology.org). Reprinted with permission.

✤ It's A Fact!!
Children As Survivors

It is a myth that children don't grieve. Children may experience the same range of feelings as adults do; the expression of that grief might be different as children have fewer tools for communicating their feelings.

Children are especially vulnerable to feelings of guilt and abandonment. It is important for them to know that the death was not their fault and that someone is there to take care of them.

Secrecy about the suicide in the hopes of protecting children may cause further complications. Explain the situation and answer children's questions honestly and with age-appropriate responses.

Source: Excerpted from "Survivors of Suicide Fact Sheet," © 2007 American Association of Suicidology (www. suicidology.org). Reprinted with permission.

What you can do:

• Listen with non-judgmental compassion

• Understand that your friend will need time to deal with their loss

• Avoid clichés

• Talk about the person who has died

• Offer practical assistance such as shopping, cooking, driving

• Find and offer information on resources, support groups, etc.

• Be aware of difficult times, like anniversaries and holidays

Where To Go For More Information

For further information, contact a community organization like the Canadian Mental Health Association (www.cmha.ca) to find out about support and resources in your community.

Chapter 29

The Stages Of Grief And Help For Recovery

The work of grief cannot be hurried. It takes a great deal of time, usually a year or more. It may be the purest pain you have ever known.

The following are stages of grief that are commonly experienced after a loss. You may not experience all of these, and you may not experience them in this order. It is important to realize, however, that what you are feeling is natural and that, with time, you will heal.

Shock

Some people experience shock after a loss, saying things like "I feel numb" and displaying no tears or emotions. Sometimes there is denial. Gradually the bereaved become aware of what has happened, and they are able to express their emotions. Other people never go through a prolonged stage of shock. They are able to express emotions immediately.

Emotional Release

At some point a person begins to feel and to hurt. It is very important not to suppress your feelings. Suppressed feelings often surface at a later time in unhealthy ways. Shared feelings are a gift, and bring a closeness to all involved.

About This Chapter: This chapter includes "The Stages of Grief," "Myths and Facts about Grief," and "Taking Care of Yourself," © Hospice of the North Shore (www.hns.org). Reprinted with permission.

Preoccupation With The Deceased Or The Crisis

Despite efforts to think of other things, a grieving person may find it difficult to shift his/her mind from thoughts about the deceased person. This is not unusual and, with time, should not be a problem.

Symptoms Of Some Physical And Emotional Distress

These distresses may come in waves. The most common physical distresses are:

- Sleeplessness;

- Tightness in the throat;

- A choking feeling;

- Shortness of breath;

- Deep sighing;

- An empty hollow feeling in the stomach;

- Lack of muscular power ("It's almost impossible to climb stairs" or "everything I lift seems heavy");

- Digestive symptoms and poor appetite.

> ✤ **It's A Fact!!**
>
> It is okay to grieve. The death of a loved one can feel like sudden, unexpected and drastic amputation of a limb without any anesthesia. The pain cannot be described and no scale can measure the loss. We want so much for our loved one to return so that we can do something, and we ache knowing that it just can't happen. You need to know that it's okay to grieve.
>
> Source: Excerpted from "When the Worst Has Happened," © 2009 by Daniel Reidenberg and SAVE. Reprinted with permission. Additional information is available at www.save.org.

Closely associated with the physical distresses may be certain emotional alternations, the most common of which are:

- A slight sense of unreality;

- Feelings of emotional distance from people—that no one really cares or understands;

- Sometimes people appear shadowy or very small;

- Sometimes there are feelings of panic, thoughts of self-destruction, or the desire to run away or "chuck it all."

These emotional disturbances can cause many people to feel they are approaching insanity, but these feelings are actually quite normal.

Hostile Reactions

You may catch yourself responding with a great deal of anger to situations that previously would not have bothered you. The feelings can be surprising and very uncomfortable. They often make people feel that they are going crazy. Anger can be directed at the doctor, the nurse, God, sometimes even at your loved one who died.

Often, there may be feelings of hurt or hostility toward family members who do not or, for various reasons cannot, provide the emotional support the grieving person may have expected from them. Anger and hostility are normal. Do not suppress your anger.

However, it is important that you understand and direct your anger towards what you are really angry at, namely the loss of someone you loved.

Guilt

There is almost always some sense of guilt in grief. The bereaved think of the many things they felt they could have done, but didn't. They accuse themselves of negligence. These hurts pop up in grief. Guilt is normal and should pass with time.

✤ It's A Fact!!

It is okay to cry. Tears release the flood of sorrow of missing the one you love. Tears relieve the brut force of hurting, enabling us to "level off" and continue our cruise along the stream of life. Shedding tears is not a sign of weakness—it is a sign of our human nature and emotions of deep despair and sorrow. It's okay to cry. It is okay to heal: We do not need to "prove" that we loved the person who has died. As the months pass we are slowly able to move around with less outward grieving each day. We need not feel "guilty", for this is not an indication that we love less. It only means that, although we don't like it, we are learning to accept death and it's finality of the pain our loved one suffered. It's a healthy sign of healing. It's okay to heal.

Source: Excerpted from "When the Worst Has Happened," © 2009 by Daniel Reidenberg and SAVE. Reprinted with permission. Additional information is available at www .save.org.

Depression

Many grieving people feel total despair, unbearable loneliness and hopelessness; nothing seems worthwhile. These feelings may be even more intense for those who live alone or who have little family. These feelings are normal and should also pass with time.

Withdrawal

The grieving person often tends to withdraw from social relationships. Their daily routines are often disrupted as well. Life seems like a bad dream. This is normal and will take some effort to overcome, but the rewards are worthwhile.

♣ **It's A Fact!!**

It is okay to laugh. Laughter is not a sign of "less" grief. Laughter is not a sign of "less" love. It's a sign that many of our thoughts and memories are happy ones and our dear one would have wanted us to laugh again. It's okay to laugh.

Source: Excerpted from "When the Worst Has Happened," © 2009 by Daniel Reidenberg and SAVE. Reprinted with permission. Additional information is available at www.save.org.

Resolution And Readjustment

This comes gradually. The memories are still there, the love is still there, but the wound begins to heal. You begin to get on with life. It's hard to believe now, but you will feel better. By experiencing deep emotion and accepting it, you will grow warmth, depth, understanding and wisdom.

Myths And Facts About Grief

Myth: The pain will go away faster if you ignore it.

Fact: Trying to ignore your pain or keep it from surfacing will only make it worse in the long run. For real healing it is necessary to face your grief and actively deal with it.

Myth: It's important to be "be strong" in the face of loss.

Fact: Feeling sad, frightened or lonely is a normal reaction to loss. Crying doesn't mean you are weak. You don't need to "protect" your family or friends by putting on a brave front. Showing your true feelings can help them and you.

Myth: If you don't cry, it means you aren't sorry about the loss.

Fact: Crying is a normal response to sadness, but it's not the only one. Those who don't cry may feel the pain just as deeply as others. They may simply have other ways of showing it.

Myth: Grief should last about a year.

Fact: There is no right or wrong time frame for grieving. How long it takes can differ from person to person.

Myth: Moving on with your life means you're forgetting the one you lost.

Fact: Moving on means you've accepted your loved one's death. That is not the same as forgetting. You can create a new life and still keep your loved one's memory a part of you.

Myth: Friends can help by not bringing up the subject.

Fact: People who are grieving usually want and need to talk about their loss. Bringing up the subject can make it easier to talk about.

Taking Care Of Yourself

Though taking care of yourself seems like a luxury, it's actually essential to your health and well-being. When you're preoccupied by stress or grief, your immune system can become compromised, leading to a greater likelihood of illness. An essential component in taking care of yourself involves exercising control over your own life. You do have control over your actions, your activities and your choices. By consciously exercising that control, you gain a sense of mastery and confidence.

Use these tips to get you started in taking care of yourself:

- Laugh. Laughter, as they say, is the best medicine. It makes you forget for a while and produces endorphins, which are your body's natural way of producing pleasure.

- Get adequate rest, food and nutrition. Keeping your body energized is an important stress-buster and provides healthful benefits as well. You'll feel better physically, and soon that will translate into how you feel emotionally.

- Choose relaxing activities such as massage, yoga or meditation. Ten minutes of quiet moments can help clear your mind. Stretching your muscles through yoga will give you a sense of peace, and a massage can leave you intensely relaxed.

- Make time to do something that gives you pleasure. It doesn't have to be expensive or time-consuming to produce benefits you can feel. Listening to music, gardening, shopping, walking with a friend, or seeing a movie all provide you with the same effect.

- Join a support group. Sharing with a group of peers can help you talk through your stressful times. For some, the support from others is all they need.

- Start a journal. Writing down your feelings can be very therapeutic. It's a private venue where you can really open up.

- Consider how your faith or spirituality can provide inspiration and enlightenment. If it's important to you, going to church, even if you haven't been in awhile, may provide solace. If taking a walk on the beach gives your life meaning, then make your way to the shoreline, even if it does involve climbing a few mounds of snow to get there.

- Buy books on change, stress-relievers or self-help.

- Seek and accept help. When people offer assistance, accept it.

They might offer a suggestion that worked for them that you may have overlooked.

Every little bit helps. These tips and suggestions won't eliminate the stress but they will help reduce the negative repercussions. Some stress and anxiety is normal and it's not a bad thing, but when it starts to get progressive, that's when you should seek help. The power of time alone can motivate and clear your mind, making room for the sense of balance that so many of us desire within our demanding lifestyles.

> ✔ **Quick Tip**
>
> If you or someone you know needs help dealing with a loss call the Center for Grief and Healing at (978) 774-5100. The Center is open to anyone experiencing grief and loss, regardless of whether they've had hospice care.
>
> Source: © Hospice of the North Shore (www .hns.org).

Chapter 30

Coping With Bereavement

People React Emotionally And Physically

When coping with a death, you may go through all kinds of emotions. You may be sad, worried, or scared. You might be shocked, unprepared, or confused. You might be feeling angry, cheated, relieved, guilty, exhausted, or just plain empty. Your emotions might be stronger or deeper than usual or mixed together in ways you've never experienced before.

Some people find they have trouble concentrating, studying, sleeping, or eating when they're coping with a death. Others lose interest in activities they used to enjoy. Some people lose themselves in playing computer games or eat or drink to excess. And some people feel numb, as if nothing has happened.

All of these are normal ways to react to a death.

What Is Grief?

When we have emotional, physical, and spiritual reactions in response to a death or loss, it's known as grief or grieving. People who are grieving might:

About This Chapter: "Death and Grief," April 2007, reprinted with permission from www.kidshealth.org. Copyright © 2007 The Nemours Foundation. This information was provided by KidsHealth, one of the largest resources online for medically reviewed health information written for parents, kids, and teens. For more articles like this one, visit www .KidsHealth.org, or www.TeensHealth.org.

- feel strong emotions, such as sadness and anger;

- have physical reactions, such as not sleeping or even waves of nausea;

- have spiritual reactions to a death— for example, some people find themselves questioning their beliefs and feeling disappointed in their religion while others find that they feel more strongly than ever about their faith.

The grieving process takes time and healing usually happens gradually. The intensity of grief may be related to how sudden or predictable the loss was and how you felt about the person who died.

☞ **Remember!!**
Grief Isn't Just About Death

There are many different types of loss and not all of them are related to death. A person can also grieve over the breakup of an intimate relationship or after a parent, sibling, or friend moves away.

Source: © 2007 Nemours Foundation.

Some people write about grief happening in stages, but usually it feels more like "waves" or cycles of grief that come and go depending on what you are doing and if there are triggers for remembering the person who has died.

Different Ways Of Grieving

If you've lost someone in your immediate family, such as a parent, brother, or sister, you may feel cheated out of time you wanted to have with that person. It can also feel hard to express your own grief when other family members are grieving, too.

Some people may hold back their own grief or avoid talking about the person who died because they worry that it may make a parent or other family member sad. It's also natural to feel some guilt over a past argument or a difficult relationship with the person who died.

We don't always grieve over the death of another person. The death of a beloved pet can trigger strong feelings of grief. People may be surprised by how painful this loss can be. But the loving bonds we share with pets are real, and so are the feelings of loss and grief when they die.

All of these feelings and reactions are OK—but what can people do to get through them? How long does grief last? Will things ever get back to normal? And how will you go on without the person who has died?

Coping With Grief

Just as people feel grief in many different ways, they handle it differently, too.

Some people reach out for support from others and find comfort in good memories. Others become very busy to take their minds off the loss. Some people become depressed and withdraw from their peers or go out of the way to avoid the places or situations that remind them of the person who has died.

For some people, it can help to talk about the loss with others. Some do this naturally and easily with friends and family, while others talk to a professional therapist.

Some people may not feel like talking about it much at all because it's hard to find the words to express such deep and personal emotion or they wonder whether talking will make them feel the hurt more. This is fine, as long you find other ways to deal with your pain.

☞ Remember!!
Coping With Suicide

Losing someone to suicide can be especially difficult to deal with. People who lose friends or family members to suicide may feel intense despair and sadness because they feel unable to understand what could have led to such an extreme action. They may feel angry at the person—a completely normal emotion. Or they could feel guilty and wonder if there was something they might have done to prevent the suicide. Sometimes, after a traumatic loss, a person can become depressed and may need extra help to heal.

Source: © 2007 Nemours Foundation.

People sometimes deal with their sorrow by engaging in dangerous or self-destructive activities. Doing things like drinking, drugs, or cutting yourself to escape from the reality of a loss may seem to numb the pain, but the feeling is only temporary. This isn't really dealing with the pain, only masking it, which makes all those feelings build up inside and only prolongs the grief.

If your pain just seems to get worse, or if you feel like hurting yourself or have suicidal thoughts, tell someone you trust about how you feel.

What To Expect

It may feel like it might be impossible to recover after losing someone you love. But grief does get gradually better and become less intense as time goes by. To help get through the pain, it can help to know some of the things you might expect during the grieving process.

The first few days after someone dies can be intense, with people expressing strong emotions, perhaps crying, comforting each other, and gathering to express their support and condolences to the ones most affected by the loss. It is common to feel as if you are "going crazy" and feel extremes of anxiety, panic, sadness, and helplessness. Some people describe feeling "unreal," as if they're looking at the world from a faraway place. Others feel moody, irritable, and resentful.

Family and friends often participate in rituals that may be part of their religious, cultural, community, or family traditions, such as memorial services, wakes, or funerals. These activities can help people get through the first days after a death and honor the person who died. People might spend time together talking and sharing memories about their loved one. This may continue for days or weeks following the loss as friends and family bring food, send cards, or stop by to visit.

Many times, people show their emotions during this time. But sometimes a person can be so shocked or overwhelmed by the death that he or she doesn't show any emotion right away—even though the loss is very hard. And it's not uncommon to see people smiling and talking with others at a funeral, as if something sad had not happened. But being among other mourners can be a comfort, reminding us that some things will stay the same.

Sometimes, when the rituals associated with grieving end, people might feel like they should be "over it" because everything seems to have gone back to normal. When those who are grieving first go back to their normal activities, it might be hard to put their hearts into everyday things. Many people go back to doing regular things after a few days or a week. But although they may not talk about their loss as much, the grieving process continues.

It's natural to continue to have feelings and questions for a while after someone dies. It's also natural to begin to feel somewhat better. A lot depends on how your loss affects your life. It's OK to feel grief for days, weeks, or even longer, depending on how close you were to the person who died.

No matter how you choose to grieve, there's no one right way to do it. The grieving process is a gradual one that lasts longer for some people than others. There may be times when you worry that you'll never enjoy life the same way again, but this is a natural reaction after a loss.

Caring For Yourself

The loss of someone close to you can be stressful. It can help you to cope if you take care of yourself in certain small but important ways. Here are some that might help:

- **Remember that grief is a normal emotion:** Know that you can (and will) heal over time.

- **Participate in rituals:** Memorial services, funerals, and other traditions help people get through the first few days and honor the person who died.

- **Be with others:** Even informal gatherings of family and friends bring a sense of support and help people not to feel so isolated in the first days and weeks of their grief.

- **Talk about it when you can:** Some people find it helpful to tell the story of their loss or talk about their feelings. Sometimes a person doesn't feel like talking, and that's OK, too. No one should feel pressured to talk.

- **Express yourself:** Even if you don't feel like talking, find ways to express your emotions and thoughts. Start writing in a journal about the memories you have of the person you lost and how you're feeling since the loss. Or write a song, poem, or tribute about your loved one. You can do this privately or share it with others.

• **Exercise:** Exercise can help your mood. It may be hard to get motivated, so modify your usual routine if you need to.

• **Eat right:** You may feel like skipping meals or you may not feel hungry, but your body still needs nutritious foods.

• **Join a support group:** If you think you may be interested in attending a support group, ask an adult or school counselor about how to become involved. The thing to remember is that you don't have to be alone with your feelings or your pain.

• **Let your emotions be expressed and released:** Don't stop yourself from having a good cry if you feel one coming on. Don't worry if listening to particular songs or doing other activities is painful because it brings back memories of the person that you lost; this is common. After a while, it becomes less painful.

• **Create a memorial or tribute:** Plant a tree or garden, or memorialize the person in some fitting way, such as running in a charity run or walk (a breast cancer race, for example) in honor of the lost loved one.

Getting Help For Intense Grief

If your grief isn't letting up for a while after the death of your loved one, you may want to reach out for help. If grief has turned into depression, it's very important to tell someone.

How do you know if your grief has been going on too long? Here are some signs:

• You've been grieving for four months or more and you aren't feeling any better.

• You feel depressed.

• Your grief is so intense that you feel you can't go on with your normal activities.

☞ Remember!!
Grief After Suicide

- Know that you can survive, even if you feel you can't.

- Intense feelings of grief can be overwhelming and frightening. This is normal. You are not going crazy; you're grieving.

- Feelings of guilt, confusion, anger, and fear are common responses to grief.

- You may experience thoughts of suicide. This is common. It doesn't mean you'll act on those thoughts. However, if you begin to feel like you may, ask for help or call 911.

- Forgetfulness is a common, but temporary side effect. Grieving takes so much energy that other things may fade in importance.

- Keep asking "why" until you no longer need to ask.

- Healing takes time. Allow yourself the time you need to grieve.

- Grief has no predictable pattern or timetable. Though there are elements of commonality in grief, each person and each situation is unique.

- Delay making major decisions if possible. Selling car, quitting a job, etc. are all things that should be avoided if possible.

- The path of grief is one of twists and turns and you may often feel you are getting nowhere. Remember even setbacks are a kind of progress.

- This is the hardest thing you will ever do. Be patient with yourself. Seek out people who are willing to listen when you need to talk and who understand your need to be silent.

- Give yourself permission to seek professional help.

- Avoid people who try to tell you what to feel and how to feel it and, in particular, those who think you should "be over it by now."

- Find a support group for survivors that provides a safe place for you to express your feelings, or simply a place to go to be with other survivors who are experiencing some of the same things you're going through.

Source: "Grief After Suicide," © 2009 by Daniel Reidenberg and SAVE. Reprinted with permission. Additional information is available at www.save.org.

- Your grief is affecting your ability to concentrate, sleep, eat, or socialize as you normally do.

- You feel you can't go on living after the loss or you think about suicide, dying, or hurting yourself.

It's natural for loss to cause people to think about death to some degree. But if a loss has caused you to think about suicide or hurting yourself in some way, or if you feel that you can't go on living, it's important that you tell someone right away.

Counseling with a professional therapist can help because it allows you to talk about your loss and express strong feelings. Many counselors specialize in working with teens who are struggling with loss and depression. If you'd like to talk to a therapist and you're not sure where to begin, ask an adult or school counselor. Your doctor may also be able to recommend someone.

Will I Ever Get Over This?

Well-meaning friends and family might tell a grieving person they need to "move on" after a loss. Unfortunately, that type of advice can sometimes make people hesitate to talk about their loss, or make people think they're grieving wrong or too long, or that they're not normal. It can help to remember that the grieving process is very personal and individual—there's no right or wrong way to grieve. We all take our own time to heal.

It's important for grieving people to not drop out of life, though. If you don't like the idea of moving on, maybe the idea of "keeping on" seems like a better fit. Sometimes it helps to remind yourself to just keep on doing the best you can for now. If you feel sad, let yourself have your feelings and try not to run away from your emotions. But also keep on doing things you normally would such as being with friends, caring for your pet, working out, or doing your schoolwork.

Going forward and healing from grief doesn't mean forgetting about the person you lost. Getting back to enjoying your life doesn't mean you no longer miss the person. And how long it takes until you start to feel better isn't a measure of how much you loved the person. With time, the loving support of family and friends, and your own positive actions, you can find ways to cope with even the deepest loss.

Chapter 31

The Grieving Teen

Teen years are already tumultuous years, and the bereaved teen needs special attention. Under ordinary circumstances, teenagers go through many changes in their body image, behavior, attachments, and feelings. As they break away from their parents to develop their own identities, conflicts often arise within the family system. Life becomes even more complex when a father, mother, or other significant person dies—a shattering experience faced by one child in every ten before the age of eighteen. While people in all age groups struggle with such losses, teenagers face particularly painful adjustments following the death of a loved one.

Do teens grieve like adults?

Teens grieve deeply but often work very hard to hide their feelings. Fearing the vulnerability that comes with expression, they look for distractions rather than stay with the grief process long enough to find real relief. Feelings can be turned off quickly, much like flipping a light switch. Teens can act as if nothing has happened while they are breaking up inside. You may observe teens who take on the role of caregiver to family members or friends, in effect denying their own grief.

About This Chapter: "The Grieving Teen," is reprinted with permission from American Hospice Foundation. © 2000 American Hospice Foundation. All rights reserved. Additional information is available at American Hospice Foundation's website at www .americanhospice.org. Despite the older date of this document, the basic principles regarding the grief process in teens are still applicable.

Gender makes no distinctions when it comes to experiencing grief, but the outward signs may be different. Young men of this age may have a particularly hard time when they have been taught that showing emotion is something that girls do, but macho guys don't.

Who do teens trust and talk to?

Teens often trust only their peers, believing that no one else can understand how they feel and how they react to life's problems. Relationships with friends can be deep and meaningful, sharing conflicts occurring at home and details of their love lives.

How can adults gain the trust of teens?

To gain the trust of teens, adults must become good, nonjudgmental listeners. Let teenagers know that you are interested in them, in their views, in their ideas and thoughts. Let them know that you like and care for them. Support their ideas or gently introduce new ways to approach their ideas. Acknowledge their grief and offer your thoughts of how to ease their pain.

Does peer counseling work?

Because teens are most open to fellow teens, one approach to providing help is through peers. And it works. Peer counseling is now an elective course in many schools for teens. Peer counselors are trained to look at all kinds of life problems on a personal level and then at ways to help their peers. They are introduced to different situations that may occur, and speakers are brought in to teach them about specific topics.

Because teens are willing listen to other teens, peer counseling can play an important role in establishing communication with distressed classmates and friends, as well as steering them to professional help if it is needed. Peer counselors learn about depression, grief, communicating with parents and other adults, suicidal ideation, etc. At the same time, they learn their limitations and are assured of the support and expertise of their peer counseling teachers for consultation.

Selecting the right teacher for this is of course critical, since he or she must gain the trust and respect of the students—just as students will seek the trust and respect of the peers they may be called upon to counsel.

Do grief support groups work?

Another approach is through grief support groups, and they work, too. By sharing feelings with one another, teens find out they are not alone and that others are also struggling to rebuild shattered lives. Grief groups help teens feel understood, accepted and supported.

How do you start a group?

Decide on the format that will work best. There are three possibilities:

Opened-Ended: Using this format, new kids can arrive at any time, and group introductions will need to be made often. The advantage is that teens have more time to work on their grief, especially after sudden, violent, or traumatic deaths.

Time-Limited: These groups work best in the school setting. School schedules often do not allow the flexibility for an ongoing group. Teens may also be more comfortable knowing there is a beginning and an end to the group. The number of sessions is usually 8–12, but shorter groups could be offered along with the opportunity for teens to request an additional session or sessions.

Walk-In: This format frees the teen from any commitment and fits into the busy routine of school life. The difficulty is not knowing who or how many kids will attend.

How do you select the group members?

Group leaders have to decide on the parameters of the group. Is this going to be limited to teens who have had a parent die, or will it be more general? If there are enough teens to do a group focusing on parent loss, this type of focused group may work best. Grief groups that are broader in nature work well, too.

The Loss Inventory (see www.americanhospice.org/_articles/STUDENT LOSS INVENTORY.pdf) is a good tool in identifying bereaved teens. Other sources for referrals will come from teachers, coaches, counselors and parents. The PTA newsletter or the school web site can be a good place to advertise the group.

When should a referral to professionals be made?

It can be difficult to separate normal teen behavior from that of a grieving teen in trouble. Some of the indicators that let you know when a teen needs more than the help group or peer counselors offer are:

Dramatic Behavior Changes: A teen's home, school, and social life are the arenas for observing behavior changes. Listen and take notes if comments and concerns are being expressed.

Extraordinary Pressure: Get to know the teen and invite discussion regarding his or her activities at home or at school. Find out if keeping up with work is a problem or if the teen is feeling overwhelmed with what needs to be done. Ask if there is some time to spend alone or with friends.

Isolation: Is the teen spending too much time alone, canceling on dates and parties, or dropping out of after-school activities?

Depression: Discuss the differences between bereavement depression and clinical depression. Encourage the teen to consider further help, if indicated. Supply information about where to go to get counseling.

Death Wish: Always take any talk of dying seriously and explore the teen's thoughts and feelings on the matter. Listen carefully to messages from the teen indicating there is a death wish. When a loved one has died, it isn't uncommon to make statements such as, "I just wish I could go to sleep and not wake up in the morning," or "I don't care if I get in a car wreck." These are passive death wishes—something or someone causing a death. On the other hand, if a teen starts talking about when, where and how to do "it," or if there is a history of depression or suicidal behavior, this is a much more serious matter and needs immediate attention. Get prompt professional help.

Anger: Anger can often create problems at home, at school or with friendships. Anger needs to be expressed, but in appropriate ways. Unspoken anger can become depression. If the angry teen is creating problems, and normal ways of expression are not helping, this teen may need further counseling for anger management.

Guilt: Feelings of guilt often leave the teen isolated and alone, with an absence of self-esteem. The shame that accompanies guilt takes the form of deep, dark secrets—a very heavy weight to carry around. You can help the teen

✔ Quick Tip
What activities work with teens?

Teens will tell you that they just want to talk and not have any activities. For some grief groups this is true, but you need some ideas to fall back on if a particular group is silent and non-responsive. The following activity gets group members comfortable with each other because it immediately addresses the reason why they are there.

My Story

- The person who died in my life is _____
- The cause of death was _____
- I found out about the death when _____
- After death, I believe my loved one is _____
- My first feeling was _____ because _____
- Now I feel _____ because _____
- What makes me most angry is _____
- I worry about _____ because _____
- The hardest thing about school is _____ because _____
- My friends are _____
- The adults in my life tell me _____
- What helps me most is _____
- What helps me the least is _____

Other Ideas For Activities

- Writing or drawing spontaneously on mural paper taped to the wall
- Creating a collage using pictures and words cut from old magazines
- Constructing a book that can be used as a journal or a memory book
- Writing a poem, eulogy, or song
- Launching a balloon after writing messages to the person who died (Use biodegradable balloons and clip the string for environmental reasons.)
- Going on a field trip to a funeral home, cemetery, etc.

find some relief from these feelings by being a good listener and by not trying to talk him or her out of it. Suggest writing a letter to the person who died asking for forgiveness, perhaps even taking that letter to the grave and reading it out loud. Or list the things that are most guilt inducing on a biodegradable helium balloon and let it go. If measures like this don't help, don't hesitate to refer the teen for further therapy.

Substance Abuse: Have information about the perils of substance abuse available. There are times when teens use drugs or alcohol to try to take away the pain. Look for denial, anger and guilt with teens you suspect are using drugs or alcohol. When referring such a teen for additional help, find a therapist who specializes in grief and substance abuse.

Skipping School Or Dropping Grades: A normal part of grief is not caring about anything and a lack of motivation or interest. Help the teen understand that these intense feelings of grief are temporary, and that the more they skip school or don't do their homework, the harder it will be to catch up. Teens who are staying away from school may not know that, if this continues, they could be brought before a judge and sent to a probation home or juvenile detention center.

☞ Remember!!
Making Referrals And Offering Resources

Develop a list of mental health centers and know what services they offer. Put together a list of private therapists who specialize in adolescents, grief, substance abuse and depression. Update this list yearly.

Working with teens is both challenging and rewarding—challenging because you need to break into their world and develop a trusting relationship; rewarding because of the pleasure you will have in being a confidante to their secrets and concerns, seeing smiles and cheery greetings gradually replace those frowns and stares. Becoming a part of a teen's life as he or she struggles with life-shattering grief is a privilege to be exercised with care, but a privilege all the same.

Acting Out Sexually: The pain of grief is so great and the emptiness so profound, it is not uncommon to look for a warm body to fill the void. This closeness is usually only a temporary fix that may lead to regret, shame, and fear of disease and pregnancy. If a girl is thinking that sex will make her feel better, help her understand her displaced needs and what she may get herself into. If a boy is showing the same tendency, help him understand that the issue goes beyond contraception; what is involved is his own need to address his grief in way that will bring him real relief.

Chapter 32

Supporting A Grieving Person

It can be tough to know what to say or do when someone you care about is grieving. It's common to feel helpless, awkward, or unsure. You may be afraid of intruding, saying the wrong thing, or making the person feel even worse. Or maybe you feel there's little you can do to make things better.

While you can't take away the pain of the loss, you can provide much-needed comfort and support. There are many ways to help a grieving friend or family member, starting with letting the person know you care.

What You Need To Know About Bereavement And Grief

The death of a loved one is one of life's most difficult experiences. The bereaved struggle with many intense and frightening emotions, including depression, anger, and guilt. Often, they feel isolated and alone in their grief. Having someone to lean on can help them through the grieving process.

Don't let discomfort prevent you from reaching out to someone who is grieving. Now, more than ever, your support is needed. You might not know exactly what to say or what to do, but that's okay. You don't need to have answers or give advice. The most important thing you can do for a grieving person is to simply be there. Your support and caring presence will help them cope with the pain and begin to heal.

Understanding The Bereavement Process

The better your understanding of grief and how it is healed, the better equipped you'll be to help a bereaved friend or family member:

- There is no right or wrong way to grieve. Grief does not unfold in orderly, predictable stages. It is an emotional roller coaster, with unpredictable highs, lows, and setbacks. Everyone grieves differently, so avoid telling the bereaved what they "should" be feeling or doing.

- Grief may involve extreme emotions and behaviors. Feelings of guilt, anger, despair, and fear are common. A grieving person may yell to the heavens, obsess about the death, lash out at loved ones, or cry for hours on end. The bereaved need reassurance that what they're feeling is normal. Don't judge them or take their grief reactions personally.

- There is no set timetable for grieving. For many people, recovery after bereavement takes 18 to 24 months, but for others, the grieving process may be longer or shorter. Don't pressure the bereaved to move on or make them feel like they've been grieving too long. This can actually slow their healing.

What To Say To Someone Who Has Lost A Loved One

It is common to feel awkward when trying to comfort someone who is grieving. Many people do not know what to say or do. The following are suggestions to use as a guide.

- Acknowledge the situation. Example: "I heard that your____ died." Use the word "died." That will show that you are more open to talk about how the person really feels.

- Express your concern. Example: "I'm sorry to hear that this happened to you."

- Be genuine in your communication and don't hide your feelings. Example: "I'm not sure what to say, but I want you to know I care."

- Offer your support. Example: "Tell me what I can do for you."

- Ask how he or she feels, and don't assume you know how the bereaved person feels on any given day.

Source [of information]: American Cancer Society. [Source of text: Helpguide.org.]

✔ Quick Tip
How You Can Help Support Someone Who Is Grieving

- Let the person know you're willing to listen non-judgmentally.

- Remember there are no magic words—letting the person know you care is huge.

- Offer practical support: Shopping, errands, cooking, etc.

- Share memories you may have of the person who died.

- Support the person in exploring other available supports: Friends, faith community, a support group, therapist/counselor.

- Grief is not a linear process. Help plan for particularly trying times/dates (for example, anniversaries/ birthdays/holidays) which can re-trigger the feelings of loss.

- Remember that some things may trigger memories of loss that we can't plan for.

- Don't be afraid to have a good time or laugh together!

- Be patient. Remember that grief has no timeline. Avoid saying things like, "You should be getting on with your life."

- Share things that have been helpful to you in trying times; avoid trite consolations like: "Time heals all wounds," "At least they didn't suffer," or "I know just how you feel."

Source: "How You Can Help Support Someone Who Is Grieving," © 2009 Children's Room (www.childrensroom.org). Reprinted with permission.

Helping A Grieving Person

Listen With Compassion

Almost everyone worries about what to say to people who are grieving. But knowing how to listen is much more important. Oftentimes, well-meaning people avoid talking about the death or mentioning the deceased person. However, the bereaved need to feel that their loss is acknowledged, it's not too terrible to talk about, and their loved one won't be forgotten.

While you should never try to force someone to open up, it's important to let the bereaved know they have permission to talk about the loss. Talk candidly about the person who died and don't steer away from the subject if the deceased's name comes up. When it seems appropriate, ask sensitive questions—without being nosy—that invite the grieving person to openly express his or her feelings. Try simply asking, "Do you feel like talking?"

- Accept and acknowledge all feelings. Let the grieving person know that it's okay to cry in front of you, to get angry, or to break down. Don't try to reason with them over how they should or shouldn't feel. The bereaved should feel free to express their feelings, without fear of judgment, argument, or criticism.

- Be willing to sit in silence. Don't press if the grieving person doesn't feel like talking. You can offer comfort and support with your silent presence. If you can't think of something to say, just offer eye contact, a squeeze of the hand, or a reassuring hug.

- Let the bereaved talk about how their loved one died. People who are grieving may need to tell the story over and over again, sometimes in minute detail. Be patient. Repeating the story is a way of processing and accepting the death. With each retelling, the pain lessens.

- Offer comfort and reassurance without minimizing the loss. Tell the bereaved that what they're feeling is okay. If you've gone through a similar loss, share your own experience if you think it would help. However, don't give unsolicited advice, claim to "know" what the person is feeling, or compare your grief to theirs.

Comments To Avoid When Comforting The Bereaved

- "I know how you feel." One can never know how another may feel. You could, instead, ask your friend to tell you how he or she feels.

- "It's part of God's plan." This phrase can make people angry and they often respond with, "What plan? Nobody told me about any plan."

- "Look at what you have to be thankful for." They know they have things to be thankful for, but right now they are not important.

- "He's in a better place now." The bereaved may or may not believe this. Keep your beliefs to yourself unless asked.

- "This is behind you now; it's time to get on with your life." Sometimes the bereaved are resistant to getting on with because they feel this means "forgetting" their loved one. In addition, moving on is easier said than done. Grief has a mind of its own and works at its own pace.

- Statements that begin with "You should" or "You will." These statements are too directive. Instead you could begin your comments with: "Have you thought about..." or "You might..."

Source [of information]: American Hospice Foundation. [Source of text: Helpguide.org.]

Offer Practical Assistance

It is difficult for many grieving people to ask for help. They might feel guilty about receiving so much attention, fear being a burden, or be too depressed to reach out. You can make it easier for them by making specific suggestions—such as, "I'm going to the market this afternoon. What can I bring you from there?" or "I've made beef stew for dinner. When can I come by and bring you some?"

Consistency is very helpful, if you can manage it—being there for as long as it takes. This helps the grieving person look forward to your attentiveness without having to make the additional effort of asking again and again. You can also convey an open invitation by saying, "Let me know what I can do," which may make a grieving person feel more comfortable about asking for help. But keep in mind that the bereaved may not have the energy or motivation to call you when they need something, so it's better if you take the initiative to check in.

Be the one who takes the initiative. There are many practical ways you can help a grieving person. You can offer to:

- Shop for groceries or run errands

- Drop off a casserole or other type of food

- Help with funeral arrangements

- Stay in their home to take phone calls and receive guests

- Help with insurance forms or bills

- Take care of housework, such as cleaning or laundry

- Watch their children or pick them up from school

- Drive them wherever they need to go

- Look after their pets

- Go with them to a support group meeting

- Accompany them on a walk

- Take them to lunch or a movie

- Share an enjoyable activity (game, puzzle, art project)

Provide Ongoing Support

Grieving continues long after the funeral is over and the cards and flowers have stopped. The length of the grieving process varies from person to person. But in general, grief lasts much longer than most people expect. Your bereaved friend or family member may need your support for months or even years.

Continue your support over the long haul. Stay in touch with the grieving person, periodically checking in, dropping by, or sending letters or cards. Your support is more valuable than ever once the funeral is over, the other mourners are gone, and the initial shock of the loss has worn off.

Don't make assumptions based on outward appearances. The bereaved person may look fine on the outside, while inside he or she is suffering. Avoid saying things like "You are so strong" or "You look so well." This puts pressure on the person to keep up appearances and to hide his or her true feelings.

The pain of bereavement may never fully heal. Be sensitive to the fact that life may never feel the same. You don't "get over" the death of a loved one. The bereaved person may learn to accept the loss. The pain may lessen in intensity over time. But the sadness may never completely go away.

Offer extra support on special days. Certain times and days of the year will be particularly hard for your grieving friend or family member. Holidays, family milestones, birthdays, and anniversaries often reawaken grief. Be sensitive on these occasions. Let the bereaved person know that you're there for whatever he or she needs.

Watch For Warning Signs

It's common for a grieving person to feel depressed, confused, disconnected from others, or like they're going crazy. But if the bereaved person's symptoms don't gradually start to fade—or they get worse with time—this may be a sign that normal grief has evolved into a more serious problem, such as clinical depression.

Encourage the grieving person to seek professional help if you observe any of the following warning signs after the initial grieving period—especially if it's been over two months since the death.

- Difficulty functioning in daily life
- Extreme focus on the death
- Excessive bitterness, anger, or guilt
- Neglecting personal hygiene
- Alcohol or drug abuse
- Inability to enjoy life
- Hallucinations
- Withdrawing from others
- Constant feelings of hopelessness
- Talking about dying or suicide

It can be tricky to bring up your concerns to the bereaved person. You don't want to perceived as invasive. Instead of telling the person what to do, try stating your own feelings: "I am troubled by the fact that you aren't sleeping—perhaps you should look into getting help."

Take Talk Of Suicide Very Seriously

If a grieving friend or family member talks about suicide, get professional help right away. IN A LIFE-THREATENING EMERGENCY, CALL 911.

Supporting A Child Through Grief And Bereavement

Even very young children feel the pain of bereavement, but they learn how to express their grief by watching the adults around them. After a loss—particularly of a sibling or parent—children need support, stability, and honesty. They may also need extra reassurance that they will be cared for and kept safe. You can support children through the grieving process by demonstrating that it's okay to be sad and helping them make sense of the loss.

✔ Quick Tip
Recommendations For
Responding To Suicide Survivors

Coping with death is never easy. When suicide is the cause of death, the situation can be even more uncomfortable. Although there is no one right way to grieve a death by suicide, through experience the people of SAVE: Suicide Awareness Voices of Education (SAVE) have found the following recommendations useful and relevant.

- Understand that brain diseases such as clinical depression, anxiety disorders, bipolar illness, and schizophrenia underlie 90% of suicides.

- Depression is a no-fault disease of the brain. It is not caused just by life events such as the break-up of a relationship or loss of a job.

- Express sympathy.

- Avoid statements like, "You're you, you'll marry again." or "At least you have other children." Although well intentioned, these statements can be upsetting. A heartfelt, "I'm sorry for your loss," is appropriate.

- Understand that the survivor may be experiencing a number of intense emotions.

Answer any questions the child may have as truthfully as you can. Use very simple, honest, and concrete terms when explaining death to a child. Children, especially young children, may blame themselves for what happened and the truth helps them see they are not at fault.

Open communication will smooth the way for a child to express distressing feelings. Because children often express themselves through stories, games, and artwork, encourage this self-expression, and look for clues in those activities about how they are coping.

How To Help A Grieving Child

- Parents should allow a child, however young, to attend the funeral if he or she wants to.

- Parents should convey spiritual values about life and death, or pray with their child.

- Shock, pain, anger, bewilderment, disbelief, yearning, anxiety, depression, and stress are emotions expressed by some suicide survivors.

- Remember that grief is an intensely individualistic journey.

- Although you may have experienced grief in your life, avoid statements like, "I know how you feel." Instead ask how the person is feeling.

- Listen. Listening can be the most helpful thing you can do for a suicide survivor. Acknowledge the difficulty of the situation and be available if the survivor wants to talk.

- Find out about suicide survivor grief/support groups in your community. Many survivors have found it helpful to attend a suicide survivor support group. Encourage the survivor to attend at least three or four meetings.

- Read books about suicide. Check the SAVE Reading List (available online at http://www.save.org) for ideas. SAVE recommends *Suicide: Survivors—A Guide for Those Left Behind* by Adina Wrobleski.

Source: "Responding to Suicide Survivors," © 2009 by Daniel Reidenberg and SAVE. Reprinted with permission. Additional information is available at www.save.org.

- Meet regularly as a family to find out how everyone is coping.

- Help children find ways to symbolize and memorialize the deceased person.

- Keep the child's daily routine as normal as possible.

- Pay attention to the way a child plays; this can be one of a child's primary ways of communicating.

What Not To Do

- Don't force a child to publicly mourn if he or she doesn't want to.

- Don't give false or confusing messages, like "Grandma is sleeping now."

- Don't tell a child to stop crying because others might get upset.

- Don't try to shield a child from the loss. Children pick up on much more than adults realize. Including them in the grieving process will help them adapt and heal.

- Don't stifle your tears. By crying in front of a child, you send the message that it's okay for him or her to express feelings, too.

- Turn the child into your personal confidante; rely on another adult or a support group instead.

Chapter 33

How Suicide Affects Family Members

If This Helps

I was often told, after the suicide of my mother, that there is a gift in every tragedy. A silver lining. Such bs to most of us.

Fifteen long years later, I do have to admit I have found gifts. Gifts of courage, of strength, of sense of humor about things simply out of my control. Here are a few things that I know I handle completely differently than "before":

1. When I hear of a tragedy, a death, a diagnosis, I have no fear about picking up the phone, sending a card or grief book. Where I used to fool myself into believing the bereaved "needed space," I now know even in their self-imposed hermitude, they need to know people are with them. A simple card, e-mail, or phone message is a lot more than most know how to do.

2. When I have a medical "scare," or loss of my own, my mind's grief muscle memory goes straight through Elisabeth Kubler-Ross's stages at warp speed. I know I'll get through it. Of course, I don't skip stages and I am not automatically "through" it, but there always is that end of the tunnel

About This Chapter: This chapter begins with text from "If this helps..." by Ginny Sparrow, BA. Reprinted with permission. The chapter continues with "Sibling Grief," by Michelle Linn-Gust, © 2001. Reprinted with permission. For additional information and resources for survivors of suicide, visit http://siblingsurvivors.com or http://bereavedbysuicide.com.

light keeping me plodding along. That light was impossible to see during the first year after my mother's death. Now I know it's there, like a beacon. I can find it.

3. I take life's setbacks in stride. My poor mother didn't have the strength to get through one more rough patch and ended her life. I know I don't have that option because now that I know first hand what it does to those left behind, I could never do it myself. I know that no matter how sad and rough the times might be, there always is hope. I healed from my own mother's suicide—I can get through most anything.

4. I treat people better. I can't say I never make an inappropriate comment towards a bad driver (just ask my daughter), but boy do I feel differently now. When someone spaces out at a stop light, rather than honking my horn, I imagine that person might have had a horrible day. Perhaps he even lost someone today and is traveling in a fog. Goodness knows I drove like a moron for several months after my horrible day.

5. I don't take things personally. Iris Bolton (famed author and my support group leader—lucky me) tried to teach me that for years, but I really didn't get it. Now, I finally do. When someone hurts me, it often does say more about them than it does me. If only my mother could have had thicker skin. But because of her, I now do. Hey, a gift.

So, yes, I am strong like a bull, my skin like rubber, what you throw at me bounces off me back onto you. I can't say it still isn't hard. I can't say it still doesn't suck. But it's not the predominant thought in my mind when I think of my mother. Instead, the thought that comes to mind is me at age four. The family dog has had a litter of puppies, and my mother and I are playing with them literally for hours. Cereal for dinner that night; we had more important things to rejoice! Life, youth, playfulness, worry free afternoons. That helps.

Sibling Grief

Please Note [from the author]: The section below is a summary of some of the important aspects of sibling grief. For a more comprehensive resource, please read *Do They Have Bad Days in Heaven?*

Sibling survivors are often called the forgotten mourners. When a sibling dies, those siblings left behind, no matter their ages, are considered secondary mourners to the parents and/or if the sibling who died had a spouse and children. For those siblings still living at home, they will "lose" their parents for some time as the parents grieve the death of the deceased child. Parents can become so engrossed in their grief that they forget their living children still need reassurance they are loved and wanted. Because of the suicide, the surviving siblings' roles in the family are altered. They might feel the need to parent their parents or protect them from anything else bad happening. The opposite could also happen where the parents try to shield the living children, afraid of losing them, too.

It's estimated that 80 percent of children in the United States and Europe grow up with siblings. By approximating 1.85 children in each U.S. household (using U.S. Census statistics) and 31,000 suicides (per year), then 24,800 people become sibling survivors of suicide yearly. That means, in the past 25 years, at least 620,000 Americans became sibling survivors of suicide.

Through the life span, losing our sibling to suicide sets up complicated grief. As suicide grief is already difficult, adding in the factors relating to sibling loss reminds us of the uniqueness of the sibling bond.

✤ It's A Fact!!

People forget the importance of siblings in our lives. Listed below are some characteristics of the sibling bond:

- It's the longest relationship we'll have in our lives. We are typically only a few years apart when one is born and we become aware of each other. We usually know them longer than our parents, spouses, and children.

- We witness more life events and life changes with our siblings than anyone else.

- We share a sense of genetics, sense of family, belonging, and culture.

- They teach us how to function in society and communicate with others.

- The time spent together in our early years is greater than with our parents.

Source: From "Sibling Grief," by Michelle Linn-Gust, © 2001.

Childhood: Much of children's reactions to a sibling suicide will relate to their view of death. Some people believe children don't grieve. That's not true as children have shorter attention spans so their grief will also appear in brief periods. The grief might also manifest itself as physical pain (stomachaches, headaches, etc.) because children have underdeveloped coping skills and might not know how to express their feelings.

Adolescence: At this time, the siblings are trying to find their role in society. Each day they look in the mirror, they aren't sure who they see because they are changing so rapidly. They believe they are immortal because they don't face much death at this age. Also, adolescents are trying to separate themselves from their families but the suicide death will throw a loop in that. They will struggle with pulling away and still wanting to be hugged by their parents. At school, they might deny their grief feelings because it's easier to fit in that way.

Young Adulthood: During our early twenties to mid-forties, we continue to set our identities and carve out our lives and careers. We have lots of hope and if we lose our sibling at this time, we learn the hard way that life does not hold unlimited promises. We also experience anger that our sibling is not there for important life events like graduations, marriages, and the births of our children.

Middle Adulthood: In our mid-forties to fifties, our sacrifices become rewards as we slow down to enjoy what we have worked hard for. If our sibling dies by suicide, we might start questioning our definition of happiness and wondering if we completed what we really wanted out of life. At this time, our parents might die. If we also lose our sibling to suicide and there were unresolved issues (like disagreeing on the care of a now deceased parent, etc.), we will have to find a way to work through them alone.

Late Adulthood: After we reach our sixties, our sibling might be the only family member alive we can share memories of early life. If we lose our sibling to suicide, it will either enhance the feeling that our time to die is coming or we might not grieve because we believe we are going to die soon, too.

Typically, siblings will carry this loss through a large portion of life. We will want a way to memorialize our sibling. No one ever gets over a death, it becomes a part of us and we take it with us throughout life. Some ways we can remember our siblings include involvement in the Lifekeeper Faces of Suicide quilts, writing about our loved one, or getting involved with suicide prevention. There are many possibilities and each of us will come up with what we want to do when we are ready.

Part Five
Preventing Suicide

Chapter 34

What Is Mental Health?

Have you ever set a goal for yourself, like getting fit, making honor roll, or being picked for a team? Like lots of people, maybe you started out doing great, but then lost some of that drive and had trouble getting motivated again.

You're Not Alone

Everyone struggles with staying motivated and reaching their goals. Just look at how many people go on diets, lose weight, and then gain it back again!

The reality is that refocusing, changing, or making a new start on something, no matter how small, is a big deal. But it's not impossible. With the right approach, you can definitely do it.

Getting Motivated

So how do you stay motivated and on track with your goal? It all comes down to good planning, realistic expectations, and a stick-to-it attitude. Here's what you need to do:

About This Chapter: Text in this chapter is from "Motivation and the Power of Not Giving Up," February 2009, reprinted with permission from www.kidshealth.org. Copyright © 2009 The Nemours Foundation. This information was provided by KidsHealth, one of the largest resources online for medically reviewed health information written for parents, kids, and teens. For more articles like this one, visit www.KidsHealth.org, or www.TeensHealth.org.

First, know your goal: Start by writing down your major goal. Your major goal is the ultimate thing you'd like to see happen. For example, "I want to make honor roll," or "I want to get fit enough to make the cross-country team," or even, "I want to play in the Olympics" are all major goals because they're the final thing the goal setter wants to see happen (obviously, some goals take longer and require more work than others). It's OK to dream big. That's how people accomplish stuff. You just have to remember that the bigger the goal, the more work it takes to get there.

✎ What's It Mean?
What is mental health?

Mental health is not just the absence of mental disorder. It is defined as a state of well-being in which every individual realizes his or her own potential, can cope with the normal stresses of life, can work productively and fruitfully, and is able to make a contribution to her or his community.

In most countries, particularly low- and middle-income countries, mental health services are severely short of resources—both human and financial. Of the health care resources available, most are currently spent on the specialized treatment and care of the people with mental illness, and to a lesser extent on an integrated mental health system. Instead of providing care in large psychiatric hospitals, countries should integrate mental health into primary health care, provide mental health care in general hospitals and develop community-based mental health services.

Even less funding is available for mental health promotion, an umbrella term that covers a variety of strategies, all aimed at having a positive effect on mental health well-being in general. The encouragement of individual resources and skills, and improvements in the socioeconomic environment are among the strategies used.

Mental health promotion requires multisectoral action, involving a number of government sectors and non-governmental or community-based organizations. The focus should be on promoting mental health throughout the lifespan to ensure a healthy start in life for children and to prevent mental disorders in adulthood and old age.

Source: ""What is mental health?" http://www.who.int/features/qa/62/en/index.html. © 2007 World Health Organization. Reprinted with permission.

✔ **Quick Tip**

No Quick Fix

It often takes several attempts to achieve a goal. For example, the American Lung Association says that the average person who quits smoking tries to stop up to six times before successfully quitting for good.

Source: © 2009 Nemours Foundation.

Make it specific: It's easier to plan for and master a specific goal than a vague one. Let's say your goal is to get fit. That's pretty vague. Make it specific by defining what you want to achieve (such as muscle tone and definition or endurance), why you want to get fit, and by when. This helps you make a plan to reach your goal.

Make it realistic: People often abandon their goals because their expectations are unreasonable. Maybe they expect to get ripped abs in weeks rather than months, or to quit smoking easily after years of lighting up.

Let's say you want to run a marathon If you try to run the entire distance of 26.2 miles tomorrow without any training, you're unlikely to succeed. It takes the average person four months of training to run that far! But the bigger risk is that you'll get so bummed out that you'll give up your marathon dreams—and running—altogether.

Part of staying motivated is being realistic about what you can achieve within the timeframe you've planned. Competing on the Olympic ski team is a workable goal if you are 15 and already a star skier. But if you're 18 and only just taking your first lesson, time isn't exactly on your side.

Write it down: Put your specific goal in writing. Then write it down again. And again. Research shows that writing down a goal is part of the mental process of committing to it. Write your goal down every day to keep you focused and remind you how much you want it.

Break it down: Making any change takes self-discipline. You need to pay constant attention so you don't get sidetracked. One way to make this easier is to break a big goal into small steps. For example, let's say you want to run a marathon. If it's February and the marathon is in August, that's a realistic timeframe to prepare. Start by planning to run two miles and work up gradually to the distance you need.

Then set specific daily tasks, like eating five servings of fruit and veggies and running a certain amount a day. Put these on a calendar or planner so you can check them off. Ask a coach to help you set doable mini-goals

---

✔ Quick Tip
Five Ways To Fight Depression

If you feel depressed, it's best to do something about it—depression doesn't just go away on its own. In addition to getting help from a doctor or therapist, here are five things you can do to feel better.

Exercise: Take a 15- to 30-minute brisk walk every day—or dance, jog, or bike if you prefer. People who are depressed may not feel much like being active. But make yourself do it anyway (ask a friend to exercise with you if you need to be motivated). Once you get in the exercise habit, it won't take long to notice a difference in your mood.

In addition to getting aerobic exercise, some yoga poses can help relieve feelings of depression. Try downward-facing dog or legs-up-the-wall pose (you can find these poses on yoga websites). Two other aspects of yoga — breathing exercises and meditation—can also help people with depression feel better.

Nurture yourself with good nutrition: Depression can affect appetite. One person may not feel like eating at all, but another might overeat. If depression has affected your eating, you'll need to be extra mindful of getting the right nourishment. Proper nutrition can influence a person's mood and energy. So eat plenty of fruits and vegetables and get regular meals (even if you don't feel hungry, try to eat something light, like a piece of fruit, to keep you going).

Identify troubles, but don't dwell on them: Try to identify any situations that have contributed to your depression. When you know what's got you feeling blue and why, talk about it with a caring friend. Talking is a way to release

for additional mile amounts and for tasks to improve your performance, such as exercises to build strength and stamina so you'll stay motivated to run farther.

Reaching frequent, smaller goals is something to celebrate. It gives you the confidence, courage, and motivation to keep running—or doing whatever it is you're aiming to do. So reward yourself.

Check in with your goal: Now that you've broken your goal down into a series of mini-goals and daily tasks, check in every day.

the feelings and to receive some understanding. If there's no one to tell, pouring your heart out to a journal works just as well.

Once you air out these thoughts and feelings, turn your attention to something positive. Take action to solve problems. Ask for help if you need it. Feeling connected to friends and family can help relieve depression. (It may also help them feel there's something they can do instead of just watching you hurt.)

Express yourself: With depression, a person's creativity and sense of fun may seem blocked. By exercising your imagination (painting, drawing, doodling, sewing, writing, dancing, composing music, etc.) you not only get those creative juices flowing, you also loosen up some positive emotions. Take time to play with a friend or a pet, or do something fun for yourself. Find something to laugh about—a funny movie, perhaps. Laughter helps lighten your mood.

Look on the bright side: Depression affects a person's thoughts, making everything seem dismal, negative, and hopeless. If depression has you noticing only the negative, make an effort to notice the good things in life. Try to notice one thing, then try to think of one more. Consider your strengths, gifts, or blessings. Most of all, don't forget to be patient with yourself. Depression takes time to heal.

It helps to write down your small goals in the same way you wrote down your big goal. That way you can track what you need to do, check off tasks as you complete them, and enjoy knowing that you're moving toward your big goal.

As you accomplish a task, check it off on your list. Tell yourself, "Hey, I've run 10 miles, I'm nearly halfway to my goal!" Reward yourself with something you promised yourself when you set your goal. Feel successful—you are. Now think ahead to accomplishing the rest of your goal: "What do I have to do to reach 26 miles? How am I going to make the time to train?"

Writing down specific steps has another advantage: If you're feeling weak on willpower you can look at your list to help you refocus!

Recommit to your goal if you slip up: If you slip up, don't give up. Forgive yourself and make a plan for getting back on track.

Pat yourself on the back for everything you did right. Don't beat yourself up, no matter how far off track you get. Most people slip up when trying to make a change—it's a natural part of the process.

Writing down daily tasks and mini-goals helps here too. By keeping track of things, you'll quickly recognize when you've slipped up, making it easier to refocus and recommit to your goal. So instead of feeling discouraged, you can know exactly where you got off track and why.

What if you keep slipping up? Ask yourself if you're really committed to your goal. If you are, recommit—and put it in writing. The process of writing everything down may also help you discover when you're not really committed to a goal. For example, perhaps you're more in love with the fantasy of being a star athlete than the reality, and there's something else that you'd rather be or do.

View slip-ups as lessons and reminders of why you're trying to make a change. When you mess up, it's not a fault—it's an opportunity to learn something new about yourself. Say your goal is to fight less with your brother or sister. You may learn that it's better to say, "I can't talk about this right now" and take time to calm down when you feel your temper growing out of control.

Keep a stick-to-it attitude: Visualize yourself achieving your goal: a toned you in your prom dress or a successful you scoring the winning soccer goal. Self-visualization helps you keep what you're trying to accomplish in mind. It helps you believe it's possible. You can also call up your mental picture when willpower and motivation are low.

Positive self-talk also boosts your attitude and motivation. Tell yourself, "I deserve to make the honor roll because I've really been working hard" or "I feel great when I swim—I'm doing well on my exercise plan!"

Share with a friend: Another boost is having supportive people around you. Find a running buddy, a quit smoking buddy, or someone else with a similar goal so you can support each other. Having a goal buddy can make all the difference in times when you don't feel motivated—like getting up for that early-morning run.

If you're not getting support from someone when you really need it, you may need to take a break from that friendship and surround yourself with people who want to help you succeed. For instance, if you've been going to your friend's house to study together every Thursday after school, but now your pal is turning on the TV, IMing friends online, or gabbing on the phone and ignoring your pleas to get down to work, it's time to find another study buddy. You can't stay focused on your goal if your friend doesn't share that goal—or, even worse, is trying to hold you back. Seek out others who are on the same path you are and work with them instead.

✔ Quick Tip
Do It For Yourself

The key to making any change is to find the desire within yourself. Don't create a resolution just to please someone else or because others are telling you to change. If you're only doing something because you feel obligated to, you won't be as motivated as if you truly want it for yourself.

Source: © 2009 Nemours Foundation.

Don't Give Up

Ending an unhealthy behavior or creating a new, exciting one is all about taking responsibility for our lives. Finding the motivation to do it isn't necessarily easy, but it is always possible. You can stay motivated by writing down your goals, sticking to your schedule, and reminding yourself of what led you to set your goal in the first place. Change is exciting—we'd all be very bored without it.

Good luck in reaching your goals.

Chapter 35

Coping With Stress

Feeling like there are too many pressures and demands on you? Losing sleep worrying about tests and schoolwork? Eating on the run because your schedule is just too busy? You're not alone. Everyone experiences stress at times—adults, teens, and even kids. But there are ways to minimize stress and manage the stress that's unavoidable.

Good Stress And Bad Stress

The stress response (also called the fight or flight response) is critical during emergency situations, such as when a driver has to slam on the brakes to avoid an accident. It can also be activated in a milder form at a time when the pressure's on but there's no actual danger—like stepping up to take the foul shot that could win the game, getting ready to go to a big dance, or sitting down for a final exam. A little of this stress can help keep you on your toes, ready to rise to a challenge. And the nervous system quickly returns to its normal state, standing by to respond again when needed.

About This Chapter: "Stress," July 2007, reprinted with permission from www.kidshealth .org. Copyright © 2007 The Nemours Foundation. This information was provided by KidsHealth, one of the largest resources online for medically reviewed health information written for parents, kids, and teens. For more articles like this one, visit www.KidsHealth .org, or www.TeensHealth.org.

But stress doesn't always happen in response to things that are immediate or that are over quickly. Ongoing or long-term events, like coping with a divorce or moving to a new neighborhood or school, can cause stress, too.

Long-term stressful situations can produce a lasting, low-level stress that's hard on people. The nervous system senses continued pressure and may remain slightly activated and continue to pump out extra stress hormones over an extended period. This can wear out the body's reserves, leave a person feeling depleted or overwhelmed, weaken the body's immune system, and cause other problems.

✎ What's It Mean?

What Is Stress?

Stress is a feeling that's created when we react to particular events. It's the body's way of rising to a challenge and preparing to meet a tough situation with focus, strength, stamina, and heightened alertness.

The events that provoke stress are called stressors, and they cover a whole range of situations—everything from outright physical danger to making a class presentation or taking a semester's worth of your toughest subject.

The human body responds to stressors by activating the nervous system and specific hormones. The hypothalamus signals the adrenal glands to produce more of the hormones adrenaline and cortisol and release them into the bloodstream. These hormones speed up heart rate, breathing rate, blood pressure, and metabolism. Blood vessels open wider to let more blood flow to large muscle groups, putting our muscles on alert. Pupils dilate to improve vision. The liver releases some of its stored glucose to increase the body's energy. And sweat is produced to cool the body. All of these physical changes prepare a person to react quickly and effectively to handle the pressure of the moment.

This natural reaction is known as the stress response. Working properly, the body's stress response enhances a person's ability to perform well under pressure. But the stress response can also cause problems when it overreacts or fails to turn off and reset itself properly.

What Causes Stress Overload?

Although just enough stress can be a good thing, stress overload is a different story—too much stress isn't good for anyone. For example, feeling a little stress about a test that's coming up can motivate you to study hard. But stressing out too much over the test can make it hard to concentrate on the material you need to learn.

Pressures that are too intense or last too long, or troubles that are shouldered alone, can cause people to feel stress overload. Here are some of the things that can overwhelm the body's ability to cope if they continue for a long time:

- Being bullied or exposed to violence or injury

- Relationship stress, family conflicts, or the heavy emotions that can accompany a broken heart or the death of a loved one

- Ongoing problems with schoolwork related to a learning disability or other problems, such as ADHD (usually once the problem is recognized and the person is given the right learning support the stress disappears)

- Crammed schedules, not having enough time to rest and relax, and always being on the go

Some stressful situations can be extreme and may require special attention and care. Posttraumatic stress disorder is a very strong stress reaction that can develop in people who have lived through an extremely traumatic event, such as a serious car accident, a natural disaster like an earthquake, or an assault like rape.

Some people have anxiety problems that can cause them to overreact to stress, making even small difficulties seem like crises. If a person frequently feels tense, upset, worried, or stressed, it may be a sign of anxiety. Anxiety problems usually need attention, and many people turn to professional counselors for help in overcoming them.

Keep Stress Under Control

What can you do to deal with stress overload or, better yet, to avoid it in the first place? The most helpful method of dealing with stress is learning how to manage the stress that comes along with any new challenge, good or bad. Stress-management skills work best when they're used regularly, not just when the pressure's on. Knowing how to "de-stress" and doing it when things are relatively calm can help you get through challenging circumstances that may arise.

Here are some things that can help keep stress under control:

Take a stand against overscheduling: If you're feeling stretched, consider cutting out an activity or two, opting for just the ones that are most important to you.

Be realistic: Don't try to be perfect—no one is. And expecting others to be perfect can add to your stress level, too (not to mention put a lot of pressure on them!). If you need help on something, like schoolwork, ask for it.

Get a good night's sleep: Getting enough sleep helps keep your body and mind in top shape, making you better equipped to deal with any negative stressors. Because the biological "sleep clock" shifts during adolescence, many teens prefer staying up a little later at night and sleeping a little later in the morning. But if you stay up late and still need to get up early for school, you may not get all the hours of sleep you need.

✤ It's A Fact!!
Signs Of Stress Overload

People who are experiencing stress overload may notice some of the following signs:

- Anxiety or panic attacks

- A feeling of being constantly pressured, hassled, and hurried

- Irritability and moodiness

- Physical symptoms, such as stomach problems, headaches, or even chest pain

- Allergic reactions, such as eczema or asthma

- Problems sleeping

- Drinking too much, smoking, overeating, or doing drugs

- Sadness or depression

Everyone experiences stress a little differently. Some people become angry and act out their stress or take it out on others. Some people internalize it and develop eating disorders or substance abuse problems. And some people who have a chronic illness may find that the symptoms of their illness flare up under an overload of stress.

Learn to relax: The body's natural antidote to stress is called the relaxation response. It's your body's opposite of stress, and it creates a sense of well-being and calm. The chemical benefits of the relaxation response can be activated simply by relaxing. You can help trigger the relaxation response by learning simple breathing exercises and then using them when you're caught up in stressful situations. And ensure you stay relaxed by building time into your schedule for activities that are calming and pleasurable: reading a good book or making time for a hobby, spending time with your pet, or just taking a relaxing bath.

Treat your body well: Experts agree that getting regular exercise helps people manage stress. (Excessive or compulsive exercise can contribute to stress, though, so as in all things, use moderation.) And eat well to help your body get the right fuel to function at its best. It's easy when you're stressed out to eat on the run or eat junk food or fast food. But under stressful conditions, the body needs its vitamins and minerals more than ever. Some people may turn to substance abuse as a way to ease tension. Although alcohol or drugs may seem to lift the stress temporarily, relying on them to cope with stress actually promotes more stress because it wears down the body's ability to bounce back.

Watch what you're thinking: Your outlook, attitude, and thoughts influence the way you see things. Is your cup half full or half empty? A healthy dose of optimism can help you make the best of stressful circumstances. Even if you're out of practice, or tend to be a bit of a pessimist, everyone can learn to think more optimistically and reap the benefits.

Solve the little problems: Learning to solve everyday problems can give you a sense of control. But avoiding them can leave you feeling like you have little control and that just adds to stress. Develop skills to calmly look at a problem, figure out options, and take some action toward a solution. Feeling capable of solving little problems builds the inner confidence to move on to life's bigger ones—and it and can serve you well in times of stress.

Build Your Resilience

Ever notice that certain people seem to adapt quickly to stressful circumstances and take things in stride? They're cool under pressure and able to handle problems as they come up. Researchers have identified the qualities that make some people seem naturally resilient even when faced with high levels of stress.

If you want to build your resilience, work on developing these attitudes and behaviors:

- Think of change as a challenging and normal part of life.

- See setbacks and problems as temporary and solvable.

- Believe that you will succeed if you keep working toward your goals.

- Take action to solve problems that crop up.

- Build strong relationships and keep commitments to family and friends.

- Have a support system and ask for help.

- Participate regularly in activities for relaxation and fun.

Learn to think of challenges as opportunities and stressors as temporary problems, not disasters. Practice solving problems and asking others for help and guidance rather than complaining and letting stress build. Make goals and keep track of your progress. Make time for relaxation. Be optimistic. Believe in yourself. Be sure to breathe. And let a little stress motivate you into positive action to reach your goals.

Chapter 36

Sleep Is Vital To Your Well-Being

Sleep is food for the brain. During sleep, important body functions and brain activity occur. Skipping sleep can be harmful—even deadly, particularly if you are behind the wheel. You can look bad, you may feel moody, and you perform poorly. Sleepiness can make it hard to get along with your family and friends and hurt your scores on school exams, on the court or on the field. Remember, a brain that is hungry for sleep will get it, even when you don't expect it. For example, drowsiness and falling asleep at the wheel cause more than 100,000 car crashes every year. When you do not get enough sleep, you are more likely to have an accident, injury and/or illness.

Consequences

Not getting enough sleep or having sleep difficulties can:

- Limit your ability to learn, listen, concentrate and solve problems. You may even forget important information like names, numbers, your homework or a date with a special person in your life.

- Make you more prone to pimples. Lack of sleep can contribute to acne and other skin problems.

- Lead to aggressive or inappropriate behavior such as yelling at your

About this Chapter: "Teens and Sleep," © 2009 National Sleep Foundation (www .sleepfoundation.org). Reprinted with permission.

friends or being impatient with your teachers or family members.

- Cause you to eat too much or eat unhealthy foods like sweets and fried foods that lead to weight gain.

- Heighten the effects of alcohol and possibly increase use of caffeine and nicotine.

- Contribute to illness, not using equipment safely or driving drowsy.

Solutions

- Make sleep a priority. Decide what you need to change to get enough sleep to stay healthy, happy, and smart.

- Naps can help pick you up and make you work more efficiently, if you plan them right. Naps that are too long or too close to bedtime can interfere with your regular sleep.

- Make your room a sleep haven. Keep it cool, quiet and dark. If you need to, get eyeshades or blackout curtains. Let in bright light in the morning to signal your body to wake up.

- No pills, vitamins, or drinks can replace good sleep. Consuming caffeine close to bedtime can hurt your sleep, so avoid coffee, tea, soda/pop, and chocolate late in the day so you can get to sleep at night. Nicotine and alcohol will also interfere with your sleep.

- When you are sleep deprived, you are as impaired as driving with a blood alcohol content of .08%, which is illegal for drivers in many states. Drowsy driving causes over 100,000 crashes each year. Recognize sleep deprivation and call someone else for a ride. Only sleep can save you.

- Establish a bed and wake-time and stick to it, coming as close as you can on the weekends. A consistent sleep schedule will help you feel less tired since it allows your body to get in sync with its natural patterns. You will find that it's easier to fall asleep at bedtime with this type of routine.

- Don't eat, drink, or exercise within a few hours of your bedtime. Don't leave your homework for the last minute. Try to avoid the TV, computer and telephone in the hour before you go to bed. Stick to quiet, calm activities, and you'll fall asleep much more easily.

- If you do the same things every night before you go to sleep, you teach your body the signals that it's time for bed. Try taking a bath or shower (this will leave you extra time in the morning), or reading a book.

- Try keeping a diary or to-do lists. If you jot notes down before you go to sleep, you'll be less likely to stay awake worrying or stressing.

- When you hear your friends talking about their all-nighters, tell them how good you feel after getting enough sleep.

- Most teens experience changes in their sleep schedules. Their internal body clocks can cause them to fall asleep and wake up later. You can't change this, but you can participate in interactive activities and classes to help counteract your sleepiness. Make sure your activities at night are calming to counteract your already heightened alertness.

If teens need about 9¼ hours of sleep to do their best and naturally go to sleep around 11:00 p.m., one way to get more sleep is to start school later.

Teens' natural sleep cycle puts them in conflict with school start times. Most high school students need an alarm clock or a parent to wake them on school days. They are like zombies getting ready for school and find it hard to be alert and pay attention in class. Because they are sleep deprived, they are sleepy all day and cannot do their best.

Schools that have set later bell times find that students do not go to bed later, but get one hour more of sleep per school night, which means five hours more per week.

Enrollment and attendance improves and students are more likely to be on time when school starts. Parents and teachers report that teens are more alert in the morning and in better moods; they are less likely to feel depressed or need to visit the nurse or school counselor.

Poll Data

While everyone is accustomed to having a bad morning here and there, feeling irritable, unhappy or even sad, the National Sleep Foundation (NSF)'s 2006 Sleep in America poll found that many adolescents exhibit symptoms of a depressive mood on a frequent if not daily basis, and these teens are more likely to have sleep problems.

The NSF poll calculated depressive mood scores for each of the 1,602 poll respondents by measuring adolescents' responses to four mood states (using a scale of "one" to "three" where one equals "not at all" and three equals "much"):

• Felt unhappy, sad or depressed

• Felt hopeless about the future

• Felt nervous or tense

• Worried too much about things

The results showed that about half (46%) of the adolescents surveyed had a depressive mood score of 10 to 14, 37% had a score of 15 to 19, and 17% had a score of 20 to 30; these scores are considered low, moderate and high respectively.

Most notably, those adolescents with high scores ranging from 20 to 30 were more likely than those with lower scores to take longer to fall asleep on school nights, get an insufficient amount of sleep and have sleep problems related to sleepiness. In fact, 73% of those adolescents who report feeling unhappy, sad, or depressed also report not getting enough sleep at night and being excessively sleepy during the day.

While many adults may think that adolescents have things easy or don't have much to worry about—the opposite seems true according to the NSF poll. Most adolescents were likely to say they worried about things too much (58%) and/or felt stressed out/anxious (56%). Many of the adolescents surveyed also reported feeling hopeless about the future, or feeling unhappy, sad or depressed much or somewhat within the past two weeks of surveying.

Research shows that lack of sleep affects mood, and a depressed mood can lead to lack of sleep. To combat this vicious cycle, sleep experts recommend that teens prioritize sleep and focus on healthy sleep habits. Teens can start by getting the 8.5 to 9.25 hours of sleep they need each night, keeping consistent sleep and wake schedules on school nights and weekends, and opting for relaxing activities such as reading or taking a warm shower or bath before bed instead of turning on the TV or computer.

"If parents and teens know what good sleep entails and the benefits of making and sticking to a plan that supports good sleep, then they might re-examine their choices about what truly are their 'essential' activities," says Mary Carskadon, Ph.D., Director of Chronobiology/Sleep Research at the E.P. Bradley Hospital and Professor of Psychiatry and Human Behavior at Brown Medical School in Providence, Rhode Island. "The earlier parents can start helping their children with good sleep habits, the easier it will be to sustain them through the teen years."

Chapter 37

Body Image And Self-Esteem

I'm fat. I'm too skinny. I'd be happy if I were taller, shorter, had curly hair, straight hair, a smaller nose, bigger muscles, longer legs.

Do any of these statements sound familiar? Are you used to putting yourself down? If so, you're not alone. As a teen, you're going through a ton of changes in your body. And as your body changes, so does your image of yourself. Lots of people have trouble adjusting, and this can affect their self-esteem.

Why Are Self-Esteem And Body Image Important?

Self-esteem is all about how much people value themselves, the pride they feel in themselves, and how worthwhile they feel. Self-esteem is important because feeling good about yourself can affect how you act. A person who has high self-esteem will make friends easily, is more in control of his or her behavior, and will enjoy life more.

Body image is how someone feels about his or her own physical appearance.

For many people, especially those in their early teens, body image can be closely linked to self-esteem. That's because as kids develop into teens, they care more about how others see them.

About This Chapter: "Body Image And Self-Esteem," May 2009, reprinted with permission from www.kidshealth.org. Copyright © 2009 The Nemours Foundation. This information was provided by KidsHealth, one of the largest resources online for medically reviewed health information written for parents, kids, and teens. For more articles like this one, visit www.KidsHealth.org, or www.TeensHealth.org.

What Influences A Person's Self-Esteem?

Puberty: Some teens struggle with their self-esteem when they begin puberty because the body goes through many changes. These changes, combined with a natural desire to feel accepted, mean it can be tempting for people to compare themselves with others. They may compare themselves with the people around them or with actors and celebs they see on TV, in movies, or in magazines.

But it's impossible to measure ourselves against others because the changes that come with puberty are different for everyone. Some people start developing early; others are late bloomers. Some get a temporary layer of fat to prepare for a growth spurt, others fill out permanently, and others feel like they stay skinny no matter how much they eat. It all depends on how our genes have programmed our bodies to act.

The changes that come with puberty can affect how both girls and guys feel about themselves. Some girls may feel uncomfortable or embarrassed about their maturing bodies. Others may wish that they were developing faster. Girls may feel pressure to be thin but guys may feel like they don't look big or muscular enough.

Outside Influences: It's not just development that affects self-esteem, though. Many other factors (like media images of skinny girls and bulked-up guys) can affect a person's body image too.

Family life can sometimes influence self-esteem. Some parents spend more time criticizing their kids and the way they look than praising them, which can reduce kids' ability to develop good self-esteem.

People also may experience negative comments and hurtful teasing about the way they look from classmates and peers. Sometimes racial and ethnic prejudice is the source of such comments. Although these often come from ignorance, sometimes they can affect someone's body image and self-esteem.

Healthy Self-Esteem

If you have a positive body image, you probably like and accept yourself the way you are. This healthy attitude allows you to explore other aspects of growing up, such as developing good friendships, growing more independent from your parents, and challenging yourself physically and mentally. Developing these parts of yourself can help boost your self-esteem.

❖ It's A Fact!!
Resilience

People who believe in themselves are better able to recognize mistakes, learn from them, and bounce back from disappointment. This skill is called resilience.

A positive, optimistic attitude can help people develop strong self-esteem—for example, saying, "Hey, I'm human" instead of "Wow, I'm such a loser" when you've made a mistake, or not blaming others when things don't go as expected.

Knowing what makes you happy and how to meet your goals can help you feel capable, strong, and in control of your life. A positive attitude and a healthy lifestyle (such as exercising and eating right) are a great combination for building good self-esteem.

Tips For Improving Your Body Image

Some people think they need to change how they look or act to feel good about themselves. But actually all you need to do is change the way you see your body and how you think about yourself.

The first thing to do is recognize that your body is your own, no matter what shape, size, or color it comes in. If you're very worried about your weight or size, check with your doctor to verify that things are OK. But it's no one's business but your own what your body is like—ultimately, you have to be happy with yourself.

Next, identify which aspects of your appearance you can realistically change and which you can't. Everyone (even the most perfect-seeming celeb) has things about themselves that they can't change and need to accept—like their height, for example, or their shoe size.

If there are things about yourself that you want to change and can (such as how fit you are), do this by making goals for yourself. For example, if you want to get fit, make a plan to exercise every day and eat nutritious foods. Then keep track of your progress until you reach your goal. Meeting a challenge you set for yourself is a great way to boost self-esteem.

When you hear negative comments coming from within yourself, tell yourself to stop. Try building your self-esteem by giving yourself three compliments every day. While you're at it, every evening list three things in your day that really gave you pleasure. It can be anything from the way the sun felt on your face, the sound of your favorite band, or the way someone laughed at your jokes. By focusing on the good things you do and the positive aspects of your life, you can change how you feel about yourself.

Where Can I Go If I Need Help?

Sometimes low self-esteem and body image problems are too much to handle alone. A few teens may become depressed, lose interest in activities or friends—and even hurt themselves or resort to alcohol or drug abuse.

If you're feeling this way, it can help to talk to a parent, coach, religious leader, guidance counselor, therapist, or an adult friend. A trusted adult—someone who supports you and doesn't bring you down—can help you put your body image in perspective and give you positive feedback about your body, your skills, and your abilities.

If you can't turn to anyone you know, call a teen crisis hotline (check the yellow pages under social services or search online). The most important thing is to get help if you feel like your body image and self-esteem are affecting your life.

Chapter 38

Helping A Depressed Person

If someone you love has depression, you may wonder if there is anything you can do to help. The simple answer is yes. Your support and encouragement can play an important role in a loved one's recovery from depression. Yet taking care of yourself is equally important. The negativity of depression will wear you down if you don't tend to your own needs—and if it does, you won't be in a position to help your friend or family member. But with the following guidelines, you can learn how to help a depressed person while maintaining your own emotional equilibrium.

Depression is a serious but treatable disorder that affects millions of people, from young to old and from all walks of life. Depression gets in the way of everyday functioning and causes tremendous pain. And it doesn't just hurt those suffering from it—it impacts everyone around them.

If someone you love has a mood disorder, you may be struggling with any number of difficult emotions: helplessness, frustration, anger, fear, guilt, sadness. All of these feelings are normal. Dealing with a friend or family member's depression is difficult. And if you aren't careful, it can become overwhelming.

About This Chapter "Helping a Depressed Person," by Melinda Smith, M.A., Suzanne Barston, and Jeanne Segal, Ph.D., reprinted with permission from http://www.helpguide.org/mental/living_depressed_person.htm. © 2008 Helpguide.org. All rights reserved. Helpguide provides a detailed list of related references for this article, including links to information from other websites. For a complete list of Helpguide's current resources related to depression, including information about suicide and mental health, visit www.helpguide.org.

That said, you can make a difference in a friend or family member's depression by learning about the problem, encouraging treatment, and offering support. Finally, you can help by looking after your own emotional health. Taking care of yourself when someone close to you is depressed is not an act of selfishness—it's a necessity. Being emotionally strong allows you to continue to love and care for the other person.

Learning About Depression Is The First Step

Family and friends are often the first line of defense in the fight against depression. Those closest to a person with depression may notice the problem before the depressed individual does, and their influence and concern can motivate that person to seek help. But you need to understand what you're dealing with before you can help someone who is depressed, so educate yourself about its symptoms, causes, and treatment.

Signs that your friend or family member may be depressed:

• Persistently sad, irritable, or apathetic mood

• Loss of interest in normal activities

• Talking very negatively

• Withdrawing from friends and family

• Picking fights, being critical or moody

• Major change in sleeping or eating patterns

• Complaining of fatigue, lack of energy

• Frequent, unexplained aches and pains

• Having difficulties at school or work

• Abusing alcohol or drugs

The Risk Of Suicide Is Real

It may be hard to believe that the person you know and love would ever consider something as drastic as suicide, but a depressed person may not see any other way out. Depression clouds judgment and distorts thinking and can make a normally rational person believe that death is the only release from the pain he or she is feeling.

Suicide is a very real danger in depression, so it's important to know the warning signs:

- Talking about suicide, dying, or harming oneself

- Preoccupation with death

- Expressing feelings of hopelessness or self-loathing

- Acting in dangerous or self-destructive ways

♣ It's A Fact!!
Understanding Depression
In A Friend Or Family Member

- Depression is a serious condition. Don't underestimate the seriousness of depression. Depression drains a person's energy, optimism, and motivation. Your depressed loved one can't just "snap out of it" by sheer force of will.

- The symptoms of depression aren't personal. Depression makes it difficult for a person to connect on a deep emotional level with anyone, even with the person he or she loves the most. In addition, depressed people say hurtful things and lash out in anger. Remember that this is the depression talking, not your loved one, so try not to take it personally.

- Hiding the problem won't make it go away. Don't be an enabler. It doesn't help anyone involved if you are making excuses, covering up the problem, or lying for a friend or family member who is depressed. In fact, this may keep the depressed person from seeking treatment.

- You can't "fix" someone else's depression. Don't try to rescue your loved one from depression. It's not up to you to fix the problem, nor can you. You're not to blame for your loved one's depression, and you're not to feel responsible for his or her happiness (or lack thereof). Ultimately, recovery is in the hands of the depressed person.

Source: © 2008 Helpguide.org.

- Getting affairs in order and saying goodbye

- Seeking out pills, weapons, or other lethal objects

- Sudden sense of calm after a depression

If you think a friend or friend member might be considering suicide, talk to him or her about your concerns. While you may feel uncomfortable bringing up the topic, it is one of the best things you can do for a suicidal person. Talking openly about suicidal thoughts and feelings can save a life, so speak up if you're concerned and seek professional help immediately.

> **✔ Quick Tip**
>
> **What To Do In A Crisis Situation**
>
> If you believe your loved one is at an immediate risk for suicide, do NOT leave the person alone. Dial 911 or call the National Suicide Prevention Lifeline at 1-800-273-TALK.
>
> Source: © 2008 Helpguide.org.

Encouraging A Depressed Person To Get Help

Getting a depressed person into treatment can be difficult. Depression saps energy and motivation, so even the act of making an appointment or finding a doctor can seem daunting. Depression also involves negative ways of thinking. The depressed person may believe that the situation is hopeless and treatment pointless.

Because of these obstacles, getting your loved one to admit to the problem—and helping him or her see that it can be solved—is an essential step in depression recovery.

If your friend or family member resists getting help for depression:

- Suggest a general check-up with a physician. Your loved one may be less anxious about seeing a family doctor than a mental health professional. A regular doctor's visit is actually a great option, since the doctor can rule out medical causes of depression. If the doctor diagnoses depression, he or she can refer your loved one to a psychiatrist or psychologist. Sometimes, this "professional" opinion makes all the difference.

- Offer to go with the person to the family physician or to help find a new doctor or therapist. Finding the right treatment provider can be difficult, and is often a trial-and-error process. For a depressed person already low on energy, it is a huge help to have assistance making calls and looking into the options.

- Encourage your loved one to make a thorough list of symptoms and ailments to discuss with the doctor. You can even bring up things that you have noticed as an outside observer, such as, "You seem to feel much worse in the mornings," or "You always get stomach pains before work."

How To Support Someone With Depression

One of the most important things you can do to help a friend or relative with depression is to give your unconditional love and support. This involves being compassionate and patient, which is not always easy when dealing with the negativity, hostility, and moodiness that go hand in hand with depression.

Being supportive involves offering encouragement and hope. Very often, this is a matter of talking to the person in language that he or she will understand and respond to while in a depressed mindframe.

Once your friend or family member has acknowledged the depression and agreed to seek help, you can extend your support by approaching the treatment as a team effort. Offer to be involved in any way or to any degree that your loved one wants and is comfortable with. But remember that you are not—nor should you be—in the driver's seat. Defer to your loved one's wishes.

✔ **Quick Tip**
Helping A Suicidal Person
Most people who commit suicide don't want to die—they just want to stop hurting. You can help by keeping an eye out for the warning signs, speaking up about concerns, and providing reassurance and support.

Source: © 2008 Helpguide.org.

❖ It's A Fact!!
Re-Shaping Negative Thoughts Shields At-Risk Teens From Depression

At-risk teens exposed to a program that teaches them to counteract their unrealistic and overly negative thoughts experienced significantly less depression than their peers who received usual care, researchers funded by the National Institute of Mental Health (NIMH) researchers have found. However, the cognitive behavioral prevention program failed to similarly help adolescents prone to the mood disorder if their parents were currently depressed.

NIMH grantee Judy Garber, Ph.D., of Vanderbilt University, and colleagues, report on the findings of their multi-site clinical trial in the June 3, 2009 issue of the *Journal of the American Medical Association*.

Background: Only a fourth of depressed youth receive any treatment and at least 20 percent develop a chronic, difficult-to-treat form of the illness. Having a history of the illness substantially increases risk for depression, which soars two to three times among children of depressed parents. An initial study had supported the efficacy of a cognitive behavioral prevention program in reducing risk in such depression-prone teens, but it was unknown whether this would hold up across diverse "real world" settings.

To find out, Garber and Drs. David Brent, the University of Pittsburgh, William Beardslee, Boston Children's Hospital and Judge Baker Children's Center, and Gregory Clarke, Kaiser Permanente Center for Health Research in Portland, OR, randomly assigned 316 at-risk adolescents (aged 13–17) to either the cognitive behavioral program or usual care.

Teens in the cognitive behavioral program received eight weekly 90-minute group cognitive behavioral sessions. Masters or doctoral-level therapists helped them learn to restructure dysfunctional thinking patterns and practice problem solving skills. This was followed by six monthly continuation sessions in which they reviewed the cognitive and problem-solving skills and also learned relaxation, assertiveness and behavioral activation techniques.

Teens in the usual care condition as well as those in the cognitive behavior program were allowed to begin or continue with any mental health or other healthcare services available in their communities.

Results: Over a 9-month follow-up period, the rate of depression in the cognitive behavioral program group was 11 percent lower than for those in the usual care condition—21.4 percent vs. 32.7 percent. Adolescents in the prevention program also self-reported lower levels of depression symptoms than those in usual care. Among teens whose parents were not depressed at the beginning of the study, the program was more effective in preventing onset of depression than usual care—11.7 percent vs. 40.5 percent. However, this advantage did not hold for youth in the cognitive behavioral program if they had a parent who was depressed at the start of the study. Such teens had significantly higher rates of depression than those without a currently depressed parent.

Significance: The results demonstrate that the prevention program can be effectively delivered in a variety of "real world" settings, say the researchers.

"For every nine adolescents who received the cognitive intervention, we would expect to prevent one from developing a depressive episode," explained Garber. "This is comparable to what is seen with treatment response to medication."

Moreover, preventing recurrence of a depressive episode may arguably bring even greater benefits than treating an episode after it has already produced other negative consequences. This suggests that the program may be useful for maintaining recovery, once achieved, she noted.

What's Next? "Our results also underscore the link between changes in parent and youth depression. Future investigations might explore combining or sequencing parental depression and prevention programs for at-risk teens."

Reference: Prevention of depression in at-risk adolescents: a randomized controlled trial. Garber J, Clarke GN, Weersing VR, Beardslee WR, Brent DA, Gladstone TR, DeBar LL, Lynch FL, D'Angelo E, Hollon SD, Shamseddeen W, Iyengar S. JAMA. 2009 Jun 3;301(21):2215-24. PMID: 19491183

Source: From "Re-shaping Negative Thoughts Shields At-Risk Teens from Depression," a Science Update from the National Institute of Mental Health, November 2009.

Supporting The Depression Treatment Process

- Provide whatever assistance the person needs (and is willing to accept). Help him or her make and keep appointments, research treatment options, and stay on schedule with any treatment protocols.

- Have realistic expectations. It can be frustrating to watch a depressed loved one struggle, especially if progress is slow or stalled. Having patience is important. Even with optimal treatment, recovery from depression doesn't happen overnight.

- Lead by example. Encourage the depressed person to lead a healthier lifestyle by doing it yourself: maintain a positive outlook, eat better, avoid alcohol and drugs, exercise, and lean on others for support.

- Encourage activity. Invite your loved one to join you in activities that can help brighten moods, like going to a funny movie or having dinner at a favorite restaurant. Exercise is especially helpful, so try to get the depressed person out of the

---

✔ Quick Tip
Talking To A Depressed Person

What you can say that helps:

- You are not alone in this. I'm here for you.

- You many not believe it now, but the way you're feeling will change.

- I may not be able to understand exactly how you feel but I care about you and want to help.

- You are important to me. Your life is important to me.

- Tell me what I can do now to help you.

- I am here for you. We will get through this together.

What NOT to say:

- It's all in your head. Just snap out of it.

- We all go through times like these. You'll be fine.

- Look on the bright side.

- You have so much to live for; why do you want to die?

- I can't do anything about your situation.

- What's wrong with you? Shouldn't you be better by now?

Adapted from the Depression and Bipolar Support Alliance.

Source: © 2008 Helpguide.org.

house for regular walks. Be gently and lovingly persistent—don't get discouraged or stop asking.

- Pitch in when possible. Seemingly small tasks can be hard for a depressed person to manage. Offer to help out with household responsibilities or chores—but only do what you can without getting burned out yourself!

Taking Care Of Yourself While Helping A Depressed Person

There's a natural impulse to want to fix the problems of people we love, but you can't control a loved one's depression. You can, however, control how well you take care of yourself. It's just as important for you to stay healthy as it is for the depressed person to get treatment, so make your own well-being a priority.

Remember the advice of airline flight attendants: put on your own oxygen mask before you assist anyone else. In other words, make sure your own health and happiness are solid before you try to help a depressed person. You won't do your friend or family member any good if you collapse under the pressure of trying to help. But when your own needs are taken care of, you'll be in a solid place to help.

Tips For Taking Care Of Yourself

Think of this challenging time like a marathon; you need extra sustenance to keep yourself going. The following basic guidelines will help you keep up your strength as you support your loved one through depression treatment and recovery.

- Speak up for yourself. You may be hesitant to speak out when the depressed person in your life upsets you or lets you down. However, communicating will actually help the relationship in the long run. If you're suffering in silence and letting resentment build, your loved one will pick up on these negative emotions and feel even worse. Gently talk about how you're feeling before pent-up emotions make it too hard to communicate with sensitivity.

- Set boundaries. Of course you want to help, but you can only do so much. Your own health will suffer if you let your life be controlled by your loved one's depression. You can't be a caretaker round the clock without paying a psychological price. To avoid burnout and resentment, set clear limits on what you are willing and able to do. You are not your love one's therapist, so don't take on that responsibility.

- Stay on track with your own life. While some changes in your daily routine may be unavoidable while caring for your friend or relative, do your best to keep appointments and plans with friends. If your depressed loved one is unable to go on an outing or trip you had planned, ask a friend to join you instead.

- Seek support. You are NOT betraying your depressed relative or friend by turning to others for support. Joining a support group, talking to a counselor or clergyman, or confiding in a trusted friend will help you get through this tough time. You don't need to go into detail about your loved one's depression or betray confidences; instead focus on your emotions and what you are feeling. Make sure you can be totally honest with the person you turn to—no judging your emotions.

Chapter 39

Understanding And Helping A Suicidal Person

A suicidal person may not ask for help, but that doesn't mean that help isn't wanted. Most people who commit suicide don't want to die—they just want to stop hurting. Suicide prevention starts with recognizing the warning signs and taking them seriously.

If you think a friend or family member is considering suicide, you might be afraid to bring up the subject. But talking openly about suicidal thoughts and feelings can save a life. Speak up if you're concerned and seek professional help immediately! Through understanding, reassurance, and support, you can help your loved one overcome thoughts of suicide.

Understanding And Preventing Suicide

The World Health Organization estimates that approximately one million people die each year from suicide. What drives so many individuals to take their own lives? To those not in the grips of suicidal depression and despair,

About This Chapter: "Suicide Prevention," by Melinda Smith, M.A., reviewed by Jeanne Segal, Ph.D., reprinted with permission from http://www.helpguide.org/mental/suicide _prevention.htm. © 2008 Helpguide.org. All rights reserved. Helpguide provides a detailed list of related references for this article, including links to information from other websites. For a complete list of Helpguide's current resources related to suicide, including information about depression and mental health, visit www.helpguide.org.

it's difficult to understand. But a suicidal person is in so much pain that he or she can see no other option.

Suicide is a desperate attempt to escape suffering that has become unbearable. Blinded by feelings of self-loathing, hopelessness, and isolation, a suicidal person can't see any way of finding relief except through death. But despite their desire for the pain to stop, most suicidal people are deeply conflicted about ending their own lives. They wish there was an alternative to committing suicide, but they just can't see one.

♣ **It's A Fact!!**

If you're thinking about committing suicide, please read "If You're Feeling Suicidal" (available online at http://www .helpguide.org/mental/suicide_ help.htm) or call 1-800-273- TALK now!

Because of their ambivalence about dying, suicidal individuals usually give warning signs or signals of their intentions. The best way to prevent suicide is to know and watch for these warning signs and to get involved if you spot them. If you believe that a friend or family member is suicidal, you can play a role in suicide prevention by pointing out the alternatives, showing that you care, and getting a doctor or psychologist involved.

Warning Signs Of Suicide

Suicide prevention begins with an awareness of the warning signs of suicidal thoughts and feelings. Major warning signs for suicide include talking about killing or harming oneself, talking or writing a lot about death or dying, and seeking out things that could be used in a suicide attempt, such as weapons and drugs.

✔ **Quick Tip**

Take any suicidal talk or behavior seriously. It's not just a warning sign that the person is thinking about suicide—it's a cry for help.

♣ It's A Fact!!
Common Misconceptions About Suicide

FALSE: People who talk about suicide won't really do it. Almost everyone who commits or attempts suicide has given some clue or warning. Do not ignore suicide threats. Statements like "you'll be sorry when I'm dead," "I can't see any way out," —no matter how casually or jokingly said may indicate serious suicidal feelings.

FALSE: Anyone who tries to kill him/herself must be crazy. Most suicidal people are not psychotic or insane. They must be upset, grief-stricken, depressed, or despairing, but extreme distress and emotional pain are not necessarily signs of mental illness.

FALSE: If a person is determined to kill him/herself, nothing is going to stop him/her. Even the most severely depressed person has mixed feelings about death, wavering until the very last moment between wanting to live and wanting to die. Most suicidal people do not want death; they want the pain to stop. The impulse to end it all, however overpowering, does not last forever.

FALSE: People who commit suicide are people who were unwilling to seek help. Studies of suicide victims have shown that more then half had sought medical help within six month before their deaths.

FALSE: Talking about suicide may give someone the idea. You don't give a suicidal person morbid ideas by talking about suicide. The opposite is true— bringing up the subject of suicide and discussing it openly is one of the most helpful things you can do.

Source [of this information]: SAVE - Suicide Awareness Voices of Education. [Source of this text: Helpguide.org.]

A more subtle but equally dangerous warning sign of suicide is hopelessness. Studies have found that hopelessness is a strong predictor of suicide. People who feel hopeless may talk about "unbearable" feelings, predict a bleak future, and state that they have nothing to look forward to.

Other warning signs that point to a suicidal mind frame include dramatic mood swings or sudden personality changes, such as going from outgoing to withdrawn or well-behaved to rebellious. A suicidal person may also lose interest in day-to-day activities, neglect his or her appearance, and show big changes in eating or sleeping habits.

Table 39.1. Suicide Warning Signs

Talking about suicide	Any talk about suicide, dying, or self-harm. Includes statements such as "I wish I hadn't been born," "If I see you again...," "I want out," and "I'd be better off dead."
Seeking out lethal means	Looking for ways to commit suicide. Seeking access to guns, pills, knives, or other objects that could be used in a suicide attempt.
Preoccupation with death	Unusual focus on death, dying, or violence. Writing poems or stories about death.
No hope for the future	Feelings of helplessness, hopelessness, and being trapped ("There's no way out"). Belief that things will never get better or change.
Self-loathing, self-hatred	Feelings of worthlessness, guilt, shame, and self-hatred. Feeling like a burden ("Everyone would be better off without me").
Getting affairs in order	Making out a will. Giving away prized possessions. Making arrangements for family members.
Saying goodbye	Unusual or unexpected visits or calls to family and friends. Saying goodbye to people as if they won't be seen again.
Withdrawing from others	Withdrawing from friends and family. Increasing social isolation. Desire to be left alone.
Self-destructive behavior	Increased alcohol or drug use, reckless driving, unsafe sex. Taking unnecessary risks as if they have a "death wish."
Sudden sense of calm	A sudden sense of calm and happiness after being extremely depressed can mean that the person has made a decision to commit suicide.

Suicide Prevention Tips

Speak Up If You're Worried

If you spot the warning signs of suicide in someone you care about, you may wonder if it's a good idea to say anything. What if you're wrong? What if the person gets angry? Even worse, what if you plant the idea in your friend or family member's head? In such situations, it's natural to feel uncomfortable or afraid. But anyone who talks about suicide or shows other warning signs needs immediate help—the sooner the better.

✔ Quick Tip
Suicide Hotlines
To Call For Help

If you or someone you care about is suicidal, please call the National Suicide Prevention Lifeline at 1-800-273-TALK (8255) or the National Hopeline Network at 1-800-SUI-CIDE (1-800-784-2433).

These toll-free crisis hotlines offer 24-hour suicide prevention and support. Your call is free and confidential.

Talking To A Person About Suicide: If you're unsure whether someone is suicidal, the best way to find out is to ask. You can't make a person suicidal by showing that you care. In fact, giving the individual the opportunity to express his or her feelings may prevent a suicide attempt. The person may even be relieved that you brought up the issue.

Here are some questions you can ask:

- Have you ever thought that you'd be better off dead or that if you died, it wouldn't matter?

- Have you thought about harming yourself?

- Are you thinking about suicide?

Respond Quickly In A Crisis

If a friend or family member tells you that he or she is thinking about death or suicide, it's important to evaluate the immediate danger the person is in. Those at the highest risk for committing suicide in the near future have a specific suicide plan, the means to carry out the plan, a time schedule for doing it, and an intention to do it.

❖ It's A Fact!!
Level Of Suicide Risk

- **Low:** Some suicidal thoughts. No suicide plan. Says he or she won't commit suicide.

- **Moderate:** Suicidal thoughts. Vague plan that isn't very lethal. Says he or she won't commit suicide.

- **High:** Suicidal thoughts. Specific plan that is highly lethal. Says he or she won't commit suicide.

- **Severe:** Suicidal thoughts. Specific plan that is highly lethal. Says he or she will commit suicide.

The following questions can help you assess the immediate risk for suicide:

- Do you have a suicide plan?
- Do you have what you need to carry out your plan (pills, gun, etc.)?
- Do you know when you would do it?
- Do you intend to commit suicide?

If a suicide attempt seems imminent, call a local crisis center, dial 911, or take the person to an emergency room. Do not, under any circumstances, leave a suicidal person alone.

It's also wise to remove guns, drugs, knives, and other potentially lethal objects from the vicinity. In some cases, involuntary hospitalization may be necessary to keep the person safe and prevent a suicide attempt.

Offer Help And Support

If a friend or family member is suicidal, the best way to help is by offering an empathetic, listening ear. Let your loved one know that he or she is not alone and that you care. Don't take responsibility, however, for making your loved one well. You can offer support, but you can't get better for a suicidal person. He or she has to make a personal commitment to recovery.

As you're helping a suicidal person, don't forget to take care of yourself. Find someone that you trust—a friend, family member, clergyman, or counselor—to talk to about your feelings and get support of your own.

Helping A Suicidal Person

- Listen without judgment. Let a suicidal person express his or her feelings and accept those feelings without judging or discounting them. Don't act shocked, lecture on the value of life, or say that suicide is wrong.

- Offer hope. Reassure the person that help is available and that the suicidal feelings are temporary. Don't dismiss the pain he or she feels, but talk about the alternatives to suicide and let the person know that his or her life is important to you.

- Don't promise confidentiality. Refuse to be sworn to secrecy. A life is at stake and you may need to speak to a mental health professional in order to keep the suicidal person safe. If you promise to keep your discussions secret, you may have to break your word.

- Get professional help. Do everything in your power to get a suicidal person the help he or she needs. Call a crisis line for advice and referrals. Encourage the person to see a mental health professional, help locate a treatment facility, or take them to a doctor's appointment.

- Make a plan for life. Help the person develop a "Plan for Life," a set of steps he or she promises to follow during a suicidal crisis. It should include contact numbers for the person's doctor or therapist, as well as friends and family members who will help in an emergency.

✤ It's A Fact!! Antidepressants And Suicide

Overall, the risk of suicide is lower in people taking antidepressants for depression. But for some, depression medication causes an increase—rather than a decrease—in depression and suicidal thoughts and feelings. Because of this risk, the U.S. Food and Drug Administration (FDA) advises that anyone on antidepressants should be watched for increases in suicidal thoughts and behaviors. Monitoring is especially important if this is the person's first time on depression medication or if the dose has recently been changed. The risk of suicide is the greatest during the first two months of antidepressant treatment.

Risk Factors For Suicide

According to the U.S. Department of Health and Human Services, at least 90 percent of all people who commit suicide suffer from depression, alcoholism, or a combination of mental disorders. Depression in particular plays a large role in suicide. The difficulty suicidal people have imagining a solution to their suffering is due in part to the distorted thinking caused by depression.

Common suicide risk factors include:

- Mental illness
- Alcoholism or drug abuse
- Previous suicide attempts
- Family history of suicide
- Terminal illness or chronic pain
- Recent loss or stressful life event
- Social isolation and loneliness
- History of trauma or abuse

Suicide In Teens And Older Adults

In addition to the general risk factors for suicide, both teenagers and older adults are at a higher risk of suicide.

Suicide In Teens: Teenage suicide is a serious and growing problem. The teenage years can be emotionally turbulent and stressful. Teenagers face pressures to succeed and fit in. They may struggle with self-esteem issues, self-doubt, and feelings of alienation. For some, this leads to suicide. Depression is also a major risk factor for teen suicide.

Other risk factors for teenage suicide include:

• Childhood abuse

• Recent traumatic event

• Lack of a support network

• Availability of a gun

• Hostile social or school environment

• Exposure to other teen suicides

Suicide In The Elderly: The highest suicide rates of any age group occur among persons aged 65 years and older. One contributing factor is depression in the elderly that is undiagnosed and untreated.

Other risk factors for suicide in the elderly include:

• Recent death of a loved one

• Physical illness, disability, or pain

• Isolation and loneliness

• Major life changes, such as retirement

• Loss of independence

• Loss of sense of purpose

Chapter 40

Suicide Prevention: What You Can Do

How Can I "Be a Difference"?

You Can Help Your Friends

1. Use the LIFE model: **L**isten to your friends when they need to talk about problems or thoughts of suicide. **I**nsist that they be honest with you. **F**eelings, share them with each other. **E**xtend a helping hand and go with them to get a responsible adult involved to help.

2. You must remember to TLR—**T**alk, **L**isten, and **R**espond to your friends.

3. Never keep a friend's suicidal thoughts to yourself. Get a responsible adult involved immediately and encourage your friend to get professional help at once. You must be willing to risk your friendship to save your friend.

4. Encourage your friends to visit the Jason Foundation website (www .jasonfoundation.com) and visit the Pledge page. Make a promise to be there for each other in times of need.

About This Chapter: This chapter begins with "How Can I 'Be a Difference'," © The Jason Foundation, Inc. (www.jasonfoundation.com). Reprinted with permission. It continues with "How to Help Someone," © 2009 The Trevor Project (www.thetrevorproject.org). Reprinted with permission.

You Can Help Your School

1. Talk to your guidance counselor about including The Jason Foundation suicide prevention curriculum lessons in the school program (visit http://www.jason foundation.com/resources/index_programs.php for more information.)

2. Encourage your principal or guidance counselor to present a teacher staff development program for the whole faculty on the awareness and prevention of youth suicide.

3. Check to see if there is a Jason Foundation local office in your area.

4. Use youth suicide awareness and prevention as a report topic and share what you learn with others.

5. Lead a poster campaign about youth suicide prevention and display them in your school.

6. Lead a letter writing campaign to local and state legislators asking them to get involved in the awareness and prevention of the problem.

✤ It's A Fact!!

- Every 17 minutes another life is lost to suicide. Every day 86 Americans take their own life and over 1500 attempt suicide.

- Suicide is now the eighth leading cause of death in Americans.

- For every two victims of homicide in the U.S. there are three deaths from suicide.

- There are now twice as many deaths due to suicide than due to HIV/AIDS.

- More teenagers and young adults die from suicide than from cancer, heart disease, AIDS, birth defects, stroke, pneumonia and influenza, and chronic lung disease, **combined**.

- Suicide takes the lives of more than 30,000 Americans every year.

Suicide and suicidal behaviors can be reduced as the general public gains more understanding about the extent to which suicide is a problem, about the ways in which it can be prevented, and about the roles individuals and groups can play in prevention efforts.

Source: Excerpted from "Summary of National Strategy for Suicide Prevention: Goals and Objectives for Action," National Mental Health Information Center, Substance Abuse and Mental Health Services Administration, SMA01-3518, 2001.

You Can Help Your Community

1. Contact local churches and service organizations to let you share information with them about the problem of youth suicide.

2. Contact the local mall about displaying your posters about youth suicide prevention.

3. Contact your local newspaper and encourage them to publish articles that inform the public about the problem and prevention of youth suicide.

Let the Jason Foundation know the kinds of things you do in your community to help prevent youth suicide. We would like to share innovative ideas with others through our newsletter and website.

How To Help Someone

How You Can Help A Suicidal Person

*   **Listen:** Suicidal people frequently feel no one understands them, that they are not taken seriously, and that no one listens to them.

*   **Accept the person's feelings as they are:** Do not try to cheer the person up by making, positive, unrealistic statements. Do not joke about the situation.

*   **Do not be afraid to talk about suicide directly.** You will not be putting ideas into the person's head. It may, in fact, be dangerous to avoid asking a person directly if s/he is feeling suicidal.

*   **Ask them if they have developed a plan for suicide.** The presence of a well-developed plan indicates more serious intent.

*   **Remove anything dangerous** from the person's home that might be used in a suicide attempt (for example, gun, knife, razor blades, sleeping pills).

*   **Tell a trusted adult.** Do not keep it a secret. If someone you know is considering suicide, an adult is the best person to handle the situation and offer that person help. Make no deals to keep secret what a suicidal person has told you.

*   **Express your concern** for the person and your hope that the person will not choose suicide but instead will stick it out a little longer.

- Remind the person that depressed feelings do change over time.

- Point out that when death is chosen, it is final—it cannot be changed.

- Develop a plan for help with the person.

- If you cannot develop a plan and a suicide attempt is imminent, seek outside emergency help from a hospital, mental health clinic, or call "911."

Chapter 41

Preventing Suicide Contagion

Suicide Contagion Is Real

Between 1984 and 1987, journalists in Vienna covered the suicide deaths of individuals in the subway system. The coverage was extensive and dramatic. In 1987, a campaign alerted reporters to the possible negative effects of such reporting, and suggested alternate strategies for coverage. In the first six months after the campaign began, subway suicides and non-fatal attempts dropped by more than 80 percent. The total number of suicides in Vienna declined as well.

Research finds an increase in suicide by readers or viewers when the number of stories about individual suicides increases, a particular death is reported at length or in many stories, the story of an individual death by suicide is placed on the front page or at the beginning of a broadcast, or the headlines about specific suicide deaths are dramatic.

Recommendations

The media can play a powerful role in educating the public about suicide prevention. Stories about suicide can inform readers and viewers about the likely causes of suicide, its warning signs, trends in suicide rates, and recent treatment advances. They can also highlight opportunities to prevent suicide. Media stories

About This Chapter: Excerpted from "Reporting on Suicide: Recommendations for the Media," National Institute of Mental Health, 2002. Despite the older date of this document, the information about suicide contagion risks are still pertinent to today's teens.

about individual deaths by suicide may be newsworthy and need to be covered, but they also have the potential to do harm. Implementation of recommendations for media coverage of suicide has been shown to decrease suicide rates.

Certain ways of describing suicide in the news contribute to what behavioral scientists call "suicide contagion" or "copycat" suicides. Research suggests that inadvertently romanticizing suicide or idealizing those who take their own lives may encourage others to identify with the victim.

Exposure to suicide method through media reports can encourage vulnerable individuals to imitate it. Clinicians believe the danger is even greater if there is a detailed description of the method. Research indicates that detailed descriptions or pictures of the location or site of a suicide encourage imitation.

Presenting suicide as the inexplicable act of an otherwise healthy or high-achieving person may encourage identification with the victim.

♣ It's A Fact!!

Over 90 percent of suicide victims have a significant psychiatric illness at the time of their death. These are often undiagnosed, untreated, or both. Mood disorders and substance abuse are the two most common.

When both mood disorders and substance abuse are present, the risk for suicide is much greater, particularly for adolescents and young adults.

Research has shown that when open aggression, anxiety or agitation is present in individuals who are depressed, the risk for suicide increases significantly.

The cause of an individual suicide is invariably more complicated than a recent painful event such as the break-up of a relationship or the loss of a job. An individual suicide cannot be adequately explained as the understandable response to an individual's stressful occupation, or an individual's membership in a group encountering discrimination. Social conditions alone do not explain a suicide. People who appear to become suicidal in response to such events, or in response to a physical illness, generally have significant underlying mental problems, though they may be well-hidden.

Questions To Ask

- Had the victim ever received treatment for depression or any other mental disorder?
- Did the victim have a problem with substance abuse?

Angles To Pursue

- Conveying that effective treatments for most of these conditions are available (but under-utilized) may encourage those with such problems to seek help.
- Acknowledging the deceased person's problems and struggles as well as the positive aspects of his/her life or character contributes to a more balanced picture.

Interviewing Surviving Relatives And Friends

Research shows that, during the period immediately after a death by suicide, grieving family members or friends have difficulty understanding what happened. Responses may be extreme, problems may be minimized, and motives may be complicated.

Studies of suicide based on in-depth interviews with those close to the victim indicate that, in their first, shocked reaction, friends and family members may find a loved one's death by suicide inexplicable or they may deny that there were warning signs. Accounts based on these initial reactions are often unreliable.

Angles To Pursue

Thorough investigation generally reveals underlying problems unrecognized even by close friends and family members. Most victims do however give warning signs of their risk for suicide.

Some informants are inclined to suggest that a particular individual, for instance a family member, a school, or a health service provider, in some way played a role in the victim's death by suicide. Thorough investigation almost always finds multiple causes for suicide and fails to corroborate a simple attribution of responsibility.

Concerns

Dramatizing the impact of suicide through descriptions and pictures of grieving relatives, teachers or classmates or community expressions of grief may encourage potential victims to see suicide as a way of getting attention or as a form of retaliation against others.

Using adolescents on TV or in print media to tell the stories of their suicide attempts may be harmful to the adolescents themselves or may encourage other vulnerable young people to seek attention in this way.

Language

Referring to a "rise" in suicide rates is usually more accurate than calling such a rise an "epidemic," which implies a more dramatic and sudden increase than what we generally find in suicide rates.

Research has shown that the use in headlines of the word "suicide" or referring to the cause of death as "self-inflicted" increases the likelihood of contagion.

Recommendations For Language

Whenever possible, it is preferable to avoid referring to suicide in the headline. Unless the suicide death took place in public, the cause of death should be reported in the body of the story and not in the headline.

In deaths that will be covered nationally, such as of celebrities, or those apt to be covered locally, such as persons living in small towns, consider phrasing for headlines such as: "Marilyn Monroe dead at 36," or "John Smith dead at 48." Consideration of how they died could be reported in the body of the article.

In the body of the story, it is preferable to describe the deceased as "having died by suicide," rather than as "a suicide," or having "committed suicide." The latter two expressions reduce the person to the mode of death, or connote criminal or sinful behavior.

Contrasting "suicide deaths" with "non-fatal attempts" is preferable to using terms such as "successful," "unsuccessful," or "failed."

Special Situations

Celebrity Deaths

Celebrity deaths by suicide are more likely than non-celebrity deaths to produce imitation. Although suicides by celebrities will receive prominent coverage, it is important not to let the glamour of the individual obscure any mental health problems or use of drugs.

Homicide-Suicides

In covering murder-suicides be aware that the tragedy of the homicide can mask the suicidal aspect of the act. Feelings of depression and hopelessness present before the homicide and suicide are often the impetus for both.

Suicide Pacts

Suicide pacts are mutual arrangements between two people who kill themselves at the same time, and such pacts are rare. They are not the act of loving individuals who do not wish to be separated. Research shows that most pacts involve an individual who is coercive and another who is extremely dependent.

Stories To Consider Covering

- Trends in suicide rates
- Recent treatment advances
- Individual stories of how treatment was life-saving
- Stories of people who overcame despair without attempting suicide
- Myths about suicide
- Warning signs of suicide
- Actions that individuals can take to prevent suicide by others

Chapter 42

Individual, Family, And Community Connectedness Help Prevent Suicidal Behavior

Over the past three decades, scientific research and conceptual thinking have converged to suggest that suicidal behavior results from a combination of genetic, developmental, environmental, physiological, psychological, social, and cultural factors operating through diverse, complex pathways. In 2001, multiple agencies and sectors collaborated on publication of the National Strategy for Suicide Prevention, designed as a comprehensive and integrated approach to addressing suicide as a public health problem. (See Chapter 43 for more information about the National Strategy's Goals.) One of the National Strategy's primary aims is to promote opportunities and settings to enhance connectedness among persons, families, and communities.

Connectedness Between Persons

At the level of individual connectedness, a very clear pathway is that in times of stress, the number and quality of social ties people have can directly influence their access to social support—regardless of whether that support is instrumental or emotional, actual or perceived. Received or perceived social support is

About This Chapter: Text in this chapter was excerpted from "Promoting Individual, Family, and Community Connectedness to Prevent Suicidal Behavior," National Center for Injury Prevention and Control, Centers for Disease Control and Prevention, 2008. The complete document, including references, is available online at http://www.cdc.gov/ViolencePrevention.pdf/Suicide_Strategic_Direction_Full_Version-a.pdf.

hypothesized to decrease the threat-level appraisal of the experienced stress and increase a person's ability to cope with the stressful event or situation.

Close and supportive interpersonal relationships also appear to confer general psychological benefits independent of stress that increase physiologic functioning, such as cardiovascular, endocrine, and immune systems. This results in improved overall health and resistance to stress and disease. Close and supportive interpersonal relationships may also help to discourage maladaptive coping behaviors such as suicidal behaviors or substance use and by virtue of normative social influences encourage adaptive coping behaviors such as professional help-seeking.

> 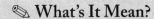 **What's It Mean?**
>
> Connectedness: Connectedness is a common thread that weaves together many of the influences of suicidal behavior and has direct relevance for suicide prevention. The Centers for Disease Control and Prevention define connectedness as the degree to which a person or group is socially close, interrelated, or shares resources with other persons or groups. This definition encompasses the nature and quality of connections both within and between multiple levels of the social ecology, including connectedness between individuals; connectedness of individuals and their families to community organizations; and connectedness among community organizations and social institutions.

Substantial evidence supports the view that connectedness between persons reduces risk of suicidal behavior. General measures of social integration (for example, number of friends, higher frequency of social contact, low levels of social isolation or loneliness) have been found to be protective against suicidal thoughts and behaviors, as documented in studies of adolescents and young and older adults.

Connectedness Of Individuals And Their Families To Community Organizations

The value of connectedness of individuals and families to community organizations has been less well studied. It nonetheless has the potential to decrease risk for suicidal behavior. Examples of relevant community organizations include schools, universities, places of employment, community centers, and churches or other religious or spiritual organizations. Connectedness of adolescents to their schools, for example, has been shown to protect against suicidal thoughts and behaviors.

Although the influence of such positive attachments on suicidal behavior needs to be better studied, many theoretical reasons support the idea that stronger connections to such groups may decrease suicidal behavior. For example, stronger connections can increase a person's sense of belonging or "mattering" to a group, a sense of personal value or worth, and access to a larger source of support. Thus persons have greater motivation and ability to cope adaptively in the face of adversity. In addition, group members often monitor each others' behavior, take responsibility for each others' well-being, and can offer or recommend assistance and support. By increasing a community's connectedness to—and responsibility for—individual members, that community is also more likely to mobilize collectively to meet its members' needs.

Connectedness Among Community Organizations And Social Institutions

In the broadest sense, connectedness among larger organizations, infrastructures, and agencies can help to prevent suicidal behavior. Although the value of stronger connections among such organizations and institutions needs improved research and understanding, schools, universities, and workplaces that use, for example, formal or informal screening strategies for suicide risk should have strong connections with agencies that can provide prevention or treatment service. Formal relationships between support services and referring organizations will help ensure not only referrals to accessible, high-quality services, but will also ensure that services are actually delivered. Moreover, better connection of helping-resource systems could promote client well-being, as in the case of the frequent disconnect between the primary health care system and the mental health care system.

❖ It's A Fact!!

Connectedness between adolescents and their parents or families has been associated with decreased suicidal behaviors. Not surprisingly, disrupted social networks (for example, family discord, problems with friends, ending of a romantic relationship) have the expected opposite effect, significantly increasing the risk of suicidal behaviors and death.

Focus On Positive Connectedness

It should be noted that the focus here is the promotion of positive (that is, health promoting, protective) connectedness. Of course, not all social connections enhance health and well-being; some research suggests that too many dependents in a person's life can lead to role overload, which can increase psychological distress. Additionally—though not yet rigorously or broadly studied—known incidents of connectedness with negative social or normative influences have allegedly contributed to suicidal behavior (for example, suicide pacts, gang involvement). These are clearly not the types of connectedness that need strengthening. They provide nonetheless clear markers of risk in which positive connectedness interventions might be most needed or most beneficial. Thus, the goal is not simply to increase the number of social ties or connections among persons or groups, but to enhance availability of and access to supportive connections.

☞ Remember!!

By supporting healthy interpersonal relationships (for example, family, peer, and marital relationships), and by encouraging communities to care about and care for their members, the population at large is likely to experience more positive health and well-being, resulting in lower risk of suicidal behavior. Further, these connections can remove social barriers to help-seeking by those in need, so persons contemplating or planning suicide would be less likely to engage in life-threatening behaviors. And if the need for social connectedness is met in a person who has engaged in nonfatal suicidal behaviors, he or she is less likely to repeat the behavior. Furthermore, following a suicide, positive social connections decrease the likelihood that survivors in the family and community will engage in suicidal behavior.

Chapter 43

Goals Of The National Strategy For Suicide Prevention

Suicide has stolen lives around the world and across the centuries. Meanings attributed to suicide and notions of what to do about it have varied with time and place, but suicide has continued to exact a relentless toll. In the United States, suicide is the eighth leading cause of death and contributes—through suicide attempts—to disability and suffering for hundreds of thousands of Americans each year. There are few who escape being touched by the tragedy of suicide in their lifetimes; those who lose someone close as a result of suicide experience an emotional trauma that may take leave, but never departs.

Only recently have the knowledge and tools become available to approach suicide as a preventable problem with realistic opportunities to save many lives. The National Strategy for Suicide Prevention: Goals and Objectives for Action (NSSP or National Strategy) is designed to be a catalyst for social change, with the power to transform attitudes, policies, and services. It reflects a comprehensive and integrated approach to reducing the loss and suffering from suicide and suicidal behaviors in the United States.

About This Chapter: Text in this chapter is excerpted from "Summary of National Strategy for Suicide Prevention: Goals and Objectives for Action," National Mental Health Information Center, Substance Abuse and Mental Health Services Administration, SMA01-3518, 2001.

❖ It's A Fact!!

As conceived, the National Strategy for Suicide Prevention (NSSP) requires a variety of organizations and individuals to become involved in suicide prevention and emphasizes coordination of resources and culturally appropriate services at all levels of government—Federal, State, tribal and community—and with the private sector. The NSSP represents the first attempt in the United States to prevent suicide through such a coordinated approach.

Because suicide is such a serious public health problem, the National Strategy proposes public health methods to address it. The public health approach to suicide prevention represents a rational and organized way to marshal prevention efforts and ensure that they are effective. Only within the last few decades has a public health approach to suicide prevention emerged with good understanding of the biological and psychosocial factors that contribute to suicidal behaviors. Its five basic steps are to clearly define the problem; identify risk and protective factors; develop and test interventions; implement interventions; and evaluate effectiveness.

Goals Of The National Strategy

Goal 1: Promote awareness that suicide is a public health problem that is preventable. In a democratic society, the stronger and broader the support for a public health initiative, the greater its chance for success. If the general public understands that suicide and suicidal behaviors can be prevented, and people are made aware of the roles individuals and groups can play in prevention, the suicide rate can be reduced.

Goal 2: Develop broad-based support for suicide prevention. Because there are many paths to suicide, prevention must address psychological, biological, and social factors if it is to be effective. Collaboration across a broad spectrum of agencies, institutions, and groups—from schools to faith-based organizations to health care associations—is a way to ensure that prevention efforts are comprehensive. Such collaboration can also generate greater and more effective attention to suicide prevention than can these groups working alone. Public/private partnerships that evolve from collaboration are able to blend resources and build upon each group's strengths. Broad-based support for suicide prevention may also lead to additional funding, through governmental programs as well as private philanthropy, and to the incorporation of suicide prevention activities into the mission of organizations that have not previously addressed it.

Goal 3: Develop and implement strategies to reduce the stigma associated with being a consumer of mental health, substance abuse, and suicide prevention services. Suicide is closely linked to mental illness and to substance abuse, and effective treatments exist for both. However, the stigma of mental illness and substance abuse prevents many persons from seeking assistance; they fear prejudice and discrimination. The stigma of suicide itself—the view that suicide is shameful and/or sinful—is also a barrier to treatment for persons who have suicidal thoughts or who have attempted suicide. Family members of suicide attempters often hide the behavior from friends and relatives, and those who have survived the suicide of a loved one suffer not only the grief of loss but often the added pain stemming from stigma. Destigmatizing mental illness and substance use disorders could increase access to treatment by reducing financial barriers, integrating care, and increasing the willingness of individuals to seek treatment.

✣ It's A Fact!!
Aims Of The National Strategy

- Prevent premature deaths due to suicide across the life span

- Reduce the rates of other suicidal behaviors

- Reduce the harmful after-effects associated with suicidal behaviors and the traumatic impact of suicide on family and friends

- Promote opportunities and settings to enhance resiliency, resourcefulness, respect, and interconnectedness for individuals, families, and communities

Goal 4: Develop and implement suicide prevention programs. Research has shown that many suicides are preventable; however, effective suicide prevention programs require commitment and resources. The public health approach provides a framework for developing preventive interventions. Programs may be specific to one particular organization, such as a university or a community health center, or they may encompass an entire state. While other goals in the NSSP address interventions to prevent suicide, a special emphasis of this goal is that of ensuring a range of interventions that in concert represent a comprehensive and coordinated program.

Goal 5: Promote efforts to reduce access to lethal means and methods of self-harm. Evidence from many countries and cultures shows that limiting access to lethal means of self-harm may be an effective strategy to prevent self-destructive behaviors. Often referred to as "means restriction," this approach is based on the belief that a small but significant minority of suicidal acts are, in fact, impulsive and of the moment; they result from a combination of psychological pain or despair coupled with the easy availability of the means by which to inflict self-injury. Thus, a self-destructive act may be prevented by limiting the individual's access to the means of self-harm. Evidence suggests that there may be a limited time effect for decreasing self-destructive behaviors in susceptible and impulsive individuals when access to the means for self-harm is restricted. Controversy exists about how to accomplish this goal because restricting means can take many forms and signifies different things to different people. For some, means restriction may connote redesigning or altering the existing lethal means of self-harm currently available, while to others it means eliminating or limiting their availability.

❖ It's A Fact!!

Historically, the stigma associated with mental illness, substance abuse, and suicide has contributed to inadequate funding for preventive services and to low insurance reimbursements for treatments. It has also resulted in the establishment of separate systems for physical health and mental health care. One consequence is that preventive services and treatment for mental illness and substance abuse are much less available than for other health problems. Moreover, this separation has led to bureaucratic and institutional barriers between the two systems that complicate the provision of services and further impede access to care.

❖ It's A Fact!!

People who regularly come into contact with individuals or families in distress need training in order to be able to recognize factors that place individuals at risk for suicide, and to learn appropriate interventions. These people, called key gatekeepers, include teachers and school personnel, clergy, police officers, primary health care providers, mental health care providers, correctional personnel, and emergency health care personnel.

Goal 6: Implement training for recognition of at-risk behavior and delivery of effective treatment. Studies indicate that many health professionals are not adequately trained to provide proper assessment, treatment, and management of suicidal patients, nor do they know how to refer clients properly for specialized assessment and treatment. Despite the increased awareness of suicide as a major public health problem, gaps remain in training programs for health professionals and others who often come into contact with patients in need of these specialized assessment techniques and treatment approaches. In addition, many health professionals lack training in the recognition of risk factors often found in grieving family members of loved ones who have died by suicide (suicide survivors).

Goal 7: Develop and promote effective clinical and professional practices: One way to prevent suicide is to identify individuals at risk and to engage them in treatments that are effective in reducing the personal and situational factors associated with suicidal behaviors (for example, depressed mood, hopelessness, helplessness, alcohol and other drug abuse, among others). Another way to prevent suicide is to promote and support the presence of protective factors, such as learning skills in problem solving, conflict resolution, and nonviolent handling of disputes. By improving clinical practices in the assessment, management, and treatment for individuals at risk for suicide, the chances for preventing those individuals from acting on their despair and distress in self-destructive ways are greatly improved. Moreover, promoting the presence of protective factors for these individuals can contribute importantly to reducing their risk.

Goal 8: Improve access to and community linkages with mental health and substance abuse services. Health disparities are attributable to differences of gender, race or ethnicity, education, income, disability, stigma, geographic location, or sexual orientation. Many of these factors place individuals at increased risk for suicidal behaviors.

Barriers to equal access and affordability of health care may be influenced by financial, structural, and personal factors. Financial barriers include not having enough health insurance or not having the financial capacity to pay for services outside a health plan or insurance program. Structural barriers include the lack of primary care providers, medical specialists or other health care professionals to meet special needs or the lack of health care facilities. Personal barriers include cultural or spiritual differences, language, not knowing when or how to seek care, or concerns about confidentiality or discrimination. Reducing disparities is a necessary step in ensuring that all Americans receive appropriate physical health, mental health, and substance abuse services. One aspect of improving access is to better coordinate the services of a variety of community institutions. This will help ensure that at-risk populations receive the services they need, and that all community members receive regular preventive health services.

Goal 9: Improve reporting and portrayals of suicidal behavior, mental illness, and substance abuse in the entertainment and news media. The media—movies, television, radio, newspapers, and magazines—have a powerful impact on perceptions of reality and on behavior. Research over many years has found that media representations of suicide may increase suicide rates, especially among youth. "Cluster suicides" and "suicide contagion" have been documented, and studies have shown that both news reports and fictional accounts of suicide in movies and on television can lead to increases in suicide. It appears that imitation plays a role in certain individuals engaging in suicidal behavior.

On the other hand, it is widely acknowledged that the media can play a positive role in suicide prevention, even as they report on suicide or depict it and related issues in movies and on television. The way suicide is presented is particularly important. Changing media representation of suicidal behaviors is one of several strategies needed to reduce the suicide rate.

Goal 10: Promote and support research on suicide and suicide prevention. All suicides are highly complex. The volume of research on suicide and its risk factors has increased considerably in the past decade and has generated new questions about why individuals become suicidal or remain suicidal. The important contributions of underlying mental illness, substance use, and biological factors, as well as potential risk that comes from certain environmental influences are becoming clearer. Increasing the understanding of how individual and environmental risk and protective factors interact with each other to affect an individual's risk for suicidal behavior is the next challenge. This understanding can contribute to the limited but growing information about how modifying risk and protective factors change outcomes pertaining to suicidal behavior.

Goal 11: Improve and expand surveillance systems. Surveillance has been defined as the systematic and ongoing collection of data. Surveillance systems are key to health planning. They are used to track trends in rates, to identify new problems, to provide evidence to support activities and initiatives, to identify risk and protective factors, to target high risk populations for interventions, and to assess the impact of prevention efforts.

Data on suicide and suicidal behavior are needed at national, state and local levels. National data can be used to draw attention to the magnitude of the suicide problem and to examine differences in rates among groups (for example, ethnic groups), locales (for example, rural vs. urban) and whether suicidal individuals were cared for in certain settings (for example, primary care, emergency departments). State and local data help establish local program priorities and are necessary for evaluating the impact of suicide prevention strategies.

✤ It's A Fact!!

Media portrayals of mental illness and substance abuse may affect the suicide rate. Negative views of these problems may lead individuals to deny they have a problem or be reluctant to seek treatment—and untreated mental illness and substance abuse are strongly correlated with suicide.

Part Six

If You Need More Information

Chapter 44

Suicide And Crisis Hot Lines

National (U.S.) Suicide Hotlines

National Suicide Hopeline
800-SUICIDE (800-784-2433)

National Suicide Prevention Lifeline
800-273-TALK (800-273-8255)

Canadian Suicide Hotline

Distress/Suicide Help Line
800-232-7288 (Canada only)

Other Toll-Free Numbers For Suicide Prevention Information

American Foundation for Suicide Prevention
888-333-AFSP (333-2377)

Jason Foundation
888-881-2323

About This Chapter: Information in this chapter was compiled from many sources deemed reliable. Inclusion does not constitute endorsement, and there is no implication associated with omission. All contact information was verified in December 2009.

Trevor Help Line
800-850-8078

Suicide Prevention Resource Center
877-GET-SPRC (438-7772)

Other Crisis Hotlines

Al-Anon/Alateen Information Line
800-344-2666
Monday through Friday, 8:00 a.m.–6:00 p.m. ET

Alcohol and Drug Help Line
WellPlace
800-821-4357

Alcohol Hotline
Adcare Hospital
800-ALCOHOL (800-252-6465)

American Council on Alcoholism
800-527-5344
10:00–6:00 p.m. MT

ARK Crisis Line
800-873-TEEN (800-873-8336)

Boys Town National Hotline
800-448-3000

Center for Substance Abuse Treatment
800-662-HELP (800-662-4357) (English)
877-767-8432 (Spanish)
800-487-4889 (TDD)

Child Quest International Sighting Line
888-818-HOPE (888-818-4673)

Mood Disorders Support Group
212-673-3000
24 Hour Hotline

NINELINE
Covenant House Hotline
800-999-9999
2:00 p.m.–12:00 a.m. ET

Eating Disorder Awareness and Prevention
National Eating Disorders Association
800-931-2237
8:30 a.m.–4:30 p.m. PT

Narconon International Help Line
800-893-7060

Emergency Shelter For Battered Women (And Their Children)
888-291-6228

NAMI Information Helpline
Nation's Voice on Mental Illness
800-950-NAMI (6264)
Monday–Friday 10:00 a.m.–6:00 p.m. ET

National Center For Missing And Exploited Children
800-THE-LOST (800-843-5678)

National Center For Victims Of Crime
800-FYI-CALL (800-394-2255)
8:30 a.m.–8:30 p.m. ET

National Child Abuse Hot Line
Childhelp USA
800-4-A-CHILD (800-422-4453)

National Clearinghouse for Alcohol and Drug Information
800-729-6686

National Domestic Violence Hot Line
800-799-7233
800-787-3224 (TTY)

National Organization for Victim Assistance
800-TRY-NOVA (800-879-6682)
Monday–Friday 9:00 a.m.–5:00 p.m. ET

National Runaway Switchboard
800-RUNAWAY (800-786-2929)
TDD: 800-621-0394

National Sexual Assault Hotline
Rape, Abuse, and Incest National Network (RAINN)
800-656-HOPE (800-656-4673)

Operation Lookout National Center For Missing Youth
800-LOOKOUT (800-566-5688)

Stop It Now!
888-PREVENT (888-773-8368)
Limited phone hours; also online at www.stopitnow.org

United Way Information Referral Service
800-233-HELP (800-233-4357)

Chapter 45

Additional Information About Suicide

Resources For Facts About Suicide And Suicide Prevention

American Association of Suicidology

5221 Wisconsin Avenue, NW
Washington, DC 20015
Phone: 202-237-2280
Fax: 202-237-2282
Website: www.suicidology.org
E-mail: info@suicidology.org

American Foundation for Suicide Prevention

120 Wall Street, 22nd Floor
New York, NY 10005
Toll-free: 888-333-AFSP
(333-2377)
Phone: 212-363-3500
Fax: 212-363-6237
Website: www.afsp.org
E-mail: inquiry@afsp.org

Feeling Blue Suicide Prevention Committee

A Non-Profit Community Service
Organization
P.O. Box 7193
St. Davids, PA 19087
Phone: 610-715-0076
Website:
http://www.feelingblue.org

About This Chapter: Information in this chapter was compiled from many sources deemed reliable. Inclusion does not constitute endorsement, and there is no implication associated with omission. All contact information was verified in December 2009.

Jason Foundation
18 Volunteer Dr.
Henderson, TN 37075
Toll-Free: 888-881-2323
Phone: 615-264-2323
Fax: 615-264-0188
Website:
http://www.jasonfoundation.com
E-mail:
info@jasonfoundation.com

Jed Foundation
220 5th Ave, 9th Floor
New York, NY 10001
Phone: 212-647-7544
Fax: 212-647-7542
Website:
http://www.jedfoundation.org
E-mail: emailus@jedfoundation.org

National Organization for People of Color Against Suicide
P.O. Box 75571
Washington, DC 20013
Toll-Free: 866-899-5317
Phone: 202-549-6039
Website: http://www.nopcas.org
E-mail: info@nopcas.org

SAVE—Suicide Awareness Voices of Education
8120 Penn Ave. S., Suite #470
Bloomington, MI 55431
Phone: 952-946-7998
Website: http://www.save.org

Suicide Prevention Action Network
1010 Vermont Ave., NW
Suite 408
Washington, DC 20005
Phone: 202-449-3600
Fax: 202-449-3601
Website: http://www.spanusa.org
E-mail: info@spanusa.org

Suicide Prevention Resource Center
55 Chapel Street
Newton, MA 02458-1060
Toll-Free: 877-GET-SPRC
(438-7772)
TTY: 617-964-5448
Website: http://www.sprc.org
E-mail: info@sprc.org

Yellow Ribbon Suicide Prevention Program
P.O. Box 644
Westminster, CO 80036
Phone: 303-429-3530
Fax: 303-426-4496
Website:
http://www.yellowribbon.org
E-mail:
ask4help@yellowribbon.org

Resources For Facts About Issues Associated With Suicide Risk

Al-Anon/Alateen Hot Line

1600 Corporate Landing Pky.
Virginia Beach, VA 23454-5617
Toll-Free: 800-344-2666
Phone: 757-563-1600
Fax: 757-563-1655
Website:
http://www.al-anon.alateen.org
E-mail: wso@al-anon.org

Association for Death Education and Counseling

111 Deer Lake Road, Suite 100
Deerfield, IL 60015
Phone: 847-509-0403
Fax: 847-480-9282
Website: www.adec.org

Centre for Addiction and Mental Health

33 Russell Street
Toronto, ON M5S 2S1
Canada
Phone: 416-535-8501
Website: http://www.camh.net

Depressed Anonymous

P.O. Box 17414
Louisville, KY 40217
Phone: 502-569-1989
Website: www.depressedanon.com
E-mail: info@depressedanon.com

Depression and Bipolar Support Alliance

730 N. Franklin St.
Suite 501
Chicago, IL 60610-7224
Toll-Free: 800-826-3632
Phone: 312-642-0049
Fax: 312-642-7243
Website:
http://www.dbsalliance.org
E-mail:
questions@dbsalliance.org

Do It Now Foundation (Drug Information)

P.O. Box 27568
Tempe, AZ 85285-7568
Phone: 480-736-0599
Fax: 480-736-0771
Website:
http://www.doitnow.org
E-mail: email@doitnow.org

Families for Depression Awareness

395 Totten Pond Road
Suite 404
Waltham, MA 02472-4808
Phone: 781-890-0220
Fax: 781-890-2411
Website: www.familyaware.org
E-mail: info@familyaware.org

National Association for Children of Alcoholics
11426 Rockville Pike, Suite 301
Rockville, MD 20852
Toll-Free: 888-55-4COAS (2627)
Phone: 301-468-0985
Fax: 301-468-0987
Website: http://www.
childrenofalcoholics.org
E-mail: nacoa@nacoa.org

National Association of Anorexia Nervosa and Associated Disorders
P.O. Box 7
Highland Park, IL 60035
Phone: 630-577-1330
Website: http://www.anad.org

National Center for Post Traumatic Stress Disorder
VA Medical Center (116D)
215 N. Main Street
White River Junction, VT 05009
Phone: 802-296-6300
Phone: 802-296-5132
Fax: 802-296-5135
Website: http://www.ncptsd.org
E-mail: ncptsd@ncptsd.org

National Center for Victims of Crime
2000 M Street NW, Suite 480
Washington, DC 20036
Phone: 202-467-8700
Fax: (202) 467-8701
Website: http://www.ncvc.org

National Center on Addiction and Substance Abuse at Columbia University
633 Third Ave., 19th Floor
New York, NY 10017-6706
Phone: 212-841-5200
Website:
http://www.casacolumbia.org

National Clearinghouse for Alcohol and Drug Information
P.O. Box 2345
Rockville, MD 20847-2345
Toll Free: 800-729-6686
Linea gratis en Español:
877-767-8432
Phone: 301-468-2600
TDD: 800-487-4889
Fax: 301-468-6433
Website: www.health.org
E-mail: info@health.org

National Coalition Against Domestic Violence
1120 Lincoln Street
Suite 1603
Denver, CO 80203
Phone: 303-839-1852
Fax: 303-831-9251
TTY: 303-839-1681
Website: http://www.ncadv.org

National Council on Alcoholism and Drug Dependence, Inc.

244 E. 58th St. 4th Floor
New York, NY 10022
Toll-Free: 800-622-2255 or
800-475-4673
Phone: 212-269-7797
Fax: 212-269-7510
Website: http://www.ncadd.org
E-mail: national@ncadd.org

National Eating Disorders Association

603 Stewart St.
Suite 803
Seattle, WA 98101
Toll Free: 800-931-2237 (hotline)
Phone: 206-382-3587
Website: http://www.
nationaleatingdisorders.org
E-mail: info@
NationalEatingDisorders.org

National Institute on Alcohol Abuse and Alcoholism

5635 Fishers Lane, MSC 9304
Bethesda, MD 20892-9304
Phone: 301-443-3860
Website: http://www.niaaa.nih.gov
E-mail:
niaaweb-r@exchange.nih.gov

National Institute on Drug Abuse

6001 Executive Boulevard
Room 5213
Bethesda, MD 20892-9561
Toll-Free: 1-800-662-HELP
(1-800-662-4357
Phone: 301-443-1124
Website: www.nida.nih.gov
E-mail: information@nida.nih.gov

National Organization for Victim Assistance

510 King Street, Suite 424
Alexandria, VA 22314
Toll-Free: 800-879-6682
Phone: 703-535-6682
Fax: 703-535-5500
Website: http://www.try-nova.org
E-mail: nova@try-nova.org

Safe and Drug-Free Schools

550 12th St. SW. 10th Floor
Washington, DC 20202-6450
Phone: 202-245-7896
Fax 202-485-0013
Website: http://www.ed.gov/offices/
OESE/SDFS
E-mail: safeschl@ed.gov

SAFE (Self-Abuse Finally Ends) Alternatives

800-DONT-CUT (800-366-8288)
Website: http://www.selfinjury.com

Samaritans of NY

P.O. Box 1259
Madison Square Station
New York, NY 10159
Suicide Prevention Hot Line:
212-673-3000
Website: http://www.samaritans
nyc.org/samhome.html

Other Mental Health Resources

American Academy of Child and Adolescent Psychiatry

3615 Wisconsin Avenue, N.W.
Washington, DC 20016-3007
Phone: 202-966-7300
Fax: 202-966-2891
Website: www.aacap.org

American Group Psychotherapy Association

25 East 21st Street
Sixth Floor
New York, NY 10010
Toll-Free: 877-668-2472
Phone: 212-477-2677
Fax: 212-979-6627
Website: http://www.agpa.org
E-mail: info@agpa.org

American Psychiatric Association

1000 Wilson Boulevard,
Suite 1825
Arlington, VA 22209-3901
Phone: 703-907-7300
Fax: 703-907-1085
E-mail: apa@psych.org
Website: www.psych.org

American Psychiatric Nurses Association

1555 Wilson Boulevard
Suite 530
Arlington, VA 22209
Toll-Free: 866-243-2443
Phone: 703-243-2443
Fax: 703-243-3390
Website: www.apna.org

American Psychological Association

750 First Street, NE
Washington, DC 20002-4242
Toll-Free: 800-374-2721
Phone: 202-336-5500
Website: www.apa.org

American Psychotherapy Association

2750 E. Sunshine Street
Springfield, MO 65804
Phone: 417-823-0173
Toll-Free: 800-205-9165
Website: www.
americanpsychotherapy.com

Anxiety Disorders Association of America

8730 Georgia Ave., Suite 600
Silver Spring, MD 20910
Phone: 240-485-1001
Fax: 240-485-1035
Website: http://www.adaa.org

Association for Behavioral and Cognitive Therapies

305 7th Avenue, 16th Floor
New York, NY 10001-60008
Phone: 212-647-1890
Fax: 212-647-1865
Website: http://www.aabt.org

Center for Mental Health Services

Substance Abuse and Mental
Health Services Administration
P.O. Box 42557
Washington, DC 20015
Rockville, MD 20847
Toll-Free: 800-789-2647
Fax: 240-221-4295
Website: mentalhealth.samhsa.gov
Mental Health Services Locator:
mentalhealth.samhsa.gov/databases

Child and Adolescent Bipolar Foundation

1000 Skokie Blvd., Suite 425
Willmette, IL 60091
Phone: 847-256-8525
Fax: 847-920-9498
Website: http://www.bpkids.org
E-mail: cabf@bpkids.org

Mood Disorders Support Group

P.O. Box 30377
New York, NY 10011
Phone: 212-533-6374
Fax: 212-675-0218
24 Hour Suicide Hotline:
212-673-3000
Website: http://www.mdsg.org
E-mail: info@mdsg.org

National Empowerment Center (Recovery from Mental Illness)

599 Canal Street, 5th Floor East
Lawrence, MA 01840
Toll-Free: 800-POWER-2-U
(800-769-3728)
Phone: 978-685-1494
Fax: 978-681-6426
Website: http://www.power2u.org
E-mail: info4@power2u.org

National Institute of Child Health and Human Development

P.O. Box 3006
Rockville, MD 20847
Toll-Free: 800-370-2943
Phone: 800-370-2943
TTY: 888-320-6942
Fax: 866-760-5947
Website: www.nichd.nih.gov
E-mail:
NICHDInformationResource
Center@mail.nih.gov

National Institute of Mental Health
6001 Executive Boulevard
Room 8184, MSC 9663
Bethesda, MD 20892-9663
Toll-Free: 866-615-NIMH
(615-6464)
Phone: 301-443-4513
TTY: 301-443-8431
Toll-Free TTY: 866-415-8051
Fax: 301-443-4279
Website: www.nimh.nih.gov
E-mail: nimhinfo@nih.gov

Obsessive Compulsive Foundation
676 State Street
New Haven, CT 06511
Phone: 203-401-2070
Fax: 203-401-2076
Website:
http://www.ocfoundation.org
E-mail: info@ocfoundation.org

Substance Abuse and Mental Health Services Administration
1 Choke Cherry Road
Rockville, MD 20857
Phone: 877-726-4727
Website: http://www.samhsa.gov

Treatment Advocacy Center
3300 N. Fairfax Drive,
Suite 220
Arlington, VA 22201
Phone: 703-294-6001
Fax: 703-294-6010
Website:
http://www.psychlaws.org
E-mail: info@psychlaws.org

Chapter 46

Resources For Suicide Survivors

Online Resources

American Association of Suicidiology

www.suicidology.org

The American Association of Suicidiology offers education, training, and suicide prevention information. Click on "Suicide Loss Survivors" for a list of resources for people who have lost someone to suicide. You can also access a directory of Suicide Survivor Support Groups at http://www.suicidology .org/web/guest/support-group-directory.

American Foundation for Suicide Prevention

http://www.afsp.org

AFSP, a non-profit organization, is involved in suicide-related research and suicide prevention. It also offers information for people whose lives have been touched by suicide. Click on "Surviving Suicide Loss" for a list of online support groups and links to additional information. Other resources for suicide survivors include a bibliography of survivor guides, personal stories, and other books written for specific audiences.

Compassionate Friends

www.compassionatefriends.org

Compassionate Friends offers help and support to grieving parents, siblings, and others following the death of a child from any cause, including suicide. The organization has chapters in all 50 states. The Compassionate Friends website includes a locator for finding a local chapter.

Department of Health (England)

http://www.dh.gov.uk

The Department of Health, a government agency in England, works with policy issues. Their publication "Help Is at Hand: A Resource for People Bereaved by Suicide and Other Sudden Traumatic Death," discusses practical matters and describes the bereavement experience. The pdf version of the booklet can be downloaded through the link at http://www.dh.gov.uk/en/ Publicationsandstatistics/Publications/PublicationsPolicyAndGuidance/ DH_087031

The Dougy Center

www.dougy.org

The Dougy Center provides structured peer support groups for children, teens, and young adults who have lost a parent, sibling, or friend as a result of suicide, homicide, accident, or illness. Information specifically written for grieving teens is available on their website at http://www.dougy.org/help/ help-for-teens.

Friends and Families of Suicides

www.pos-ffos.com

FFOS (Friends and Families of Suicides, which shares a website with Parents of Suicides) offers online support groups, memorial websites, and resources for people who have lost friends and family members by suicide. One of their projects, the Suicide Grief Support Forum, can be accessed at www .suicidegrief.com.

International Association for Suicide Prevention

www.iasp.info

The International Association for Suicide Prevention works to help prevent suicides in different cultures around the world. A directory of suicide bereavement resources is available under the "Resources" tab, and a list suicide survivor services in 18 countries can be found at www.iasp.info/resources/Postvention/Suicide_Survivor_Bereavement_Services.

Journey of Hearts

http://journeyofhearts.org

The Journey of Hearts website is designed to provide a place for people who are dealing with grief to receive support and information. A section titled "Suicide: A Complication of Grief" is available at http://journeyofhearts.org/grief/suicide.html.

The Link Counseling Center

www.thelink.org

The Link, a nonprofit counseling center, previously produced a newsletter called "The Journey" for people bereaved by suicide. Issues from 2006 and 2007 can be accessed online through a link under the tab "Suicide Prevention and Aftercare: The National Resource Center."

Suicide Prevention Action Network USA

www.spanusa.org

SPAN USA is a division of the American Foundation for Suicide Prevention. It works to influence public policy. Click on the "Survivor Support" tab to find out about connecting to other suicide survivors who want to work to reduce suicide rates across the nation.

Survivors of Suicide

www.survivorsofsuicide.com

The SOS website was designed to help people deal with suicide bereavement. Their publication "Beyond Surviving" is available at http://www.survivorsofsuicide.com/beyond_surviving.shtml.

Books

Books are listed alphabetically by title. Titles marked with an asterisk (*) were written especially for teens.

After a Suicide: Young People Speak Up*
By Susan Kuklin (Penguin Group, 1994)

Coping with Teen Suicide*
By James M. Murphy (Rosen Publishing Group, 1999)

Dying to Be Free: A Healing Guide for Families After a Suicide
By Beverly Cobain and Jean Larch (Hazeldon Publishing, 2006)

Grieving a Suicide: A Loved One's Search for Comfort, Answers and Hope
by Albert Y. Hsu (InterVarsity Press, 2002)

In Her Wake: A Child Psychiatrist Explores the Mystery of Her Mother's Suicide
By Nancy Rappaport (Basic Books, 2009)

Living When a Young Friend Commits Suicide: Or Even Starts Talking About It*
By Earl A. Grollman and Max Malikow (Beacon, 1999)

Night Falls Fast: Understanding Suicide
By Kay Redfield Jamison (Random House, 1999)

Silent Grief: Living in the Wake of Suicide (Revised Edition)
By Christopher Lucas and Henry M. Selden (Jessica Kingsley Publishers, 2007)

Suicide Index
By Joan Wickersham (Basic Books, 2009)

Touched by Suicide: Hope and Healing after Suicide
By Michael F. Myers and Carla Fine (Penguin Group, 2006)

Index

Index

Page numbers that appear in *Italics* refer to tables or illustrations. Page numbers that have a small 'n' after the page number refer to information shown as Notes at the beginning of each chapter. Page numbers that appear in **Bold** refer to information contained in boxes on that page (except Notes information at the beginning of each chapter).